CENTRAL PAIN

CENTRAL PAIN

A Neurosurgical Survey

VALENTINO CASSINARI

CARLO A. PAGNI

HARVARD UNIVERSITY PRESS

CAMBRIDGE, MASSACHUSETTS

1969

CONTENTS

CONTENTS

LIST OF FIGURES

LIST OF FIGURES

FOREWORD

It is commonly said that pain is a friendly warning stimulating man to defend himself. There are times when pain really is an alarm bell, but there are others, as Leriche said, when it is quite useless. "It is a poisoned gift. It degrades man and makes him more ill." These words of Leriche are very pertinent to the appalling pathologic situation known as central pain, in which the dominant feature in the clinical pattern is excruciating pain that is absolutely refractory to all medical treatment and that deprives the patient of rest and hope. Only surgery can, sometimes, abolish such pain. Paradoxically enough, central pain can also be the terrible complication of a surgical operation on the central nervous system designed to kill pain.

The problems of the physiopathogenesis and treatment of central pain have still not been definitively elucidated. What is worse, it is virtually impossible to foresee and avert the onset of a central pain syndrome after an antalgic operation. Central pain is thus a burning problem for the neurosurgeon, who is sometimes called upon to relieve it and at others involuntarily causes it.

The authors of this little book have gathered a great deal of data on the onset and surgical treatment of central pain in the hope that it will make some modest contribution to the knowledge and understanding of the physiopathogenesis and treatment of this condition. For this reason I feel sure that the study will be welcomed by all those who have to face the arduous problem of how to deal with intractable pain.

Paolo E. Maspes

Milan
December 1968

CENTRAL PAIN

INTRODUCTION

The problem of pain in lesions of the central nervous system was explored many years ago by Déjerine and Roussy (1906), Garcin (1937), Ajuraguerra (1937), and Riddoch and Critchley (1937). Basing their studies on spontaneous lesions of the nervous system that had given rise to pain, these workers sought to interpret "pains of central origin" in physiopathological terms. These studies yielded data of great interest. But because spontaneous lesions are usually extensive and affect many functional systems, they do not generally admit of a straight physiopathological interpretation and thus workers in this field have reached different —sometimes conflicting—conclusions in their effort to identify the structures affected by lesions causing the onset of central pain.

In the recent literature there have been many, though mainly isolated, accounts of central pain arising after surgical operations on the central nervous system, most of which had been designed to suppress pain. These observations, especially when supported by necropsy findings and by careful clinical study, are, we feel, of great importance. The lesions were made in predetermined structures, were generally circumscribed, and were, in the main, unaccompanied by the collateral phenomena that are so frequent in spontaneous lesions. They thus rank in a sense as "experimental lesions." Although the first observations of this type date back to the early 1900's, there is, as far as we know, no work in the literature that collects all these data and attempts a restatement of the physiopathological mechanisms underlying central pain. We therefore thought it would be of interest to gather all the cases so far described in the literature, especially since knowledge of the physiological anatomy of the systems

1

mediating the transmission and elaboration of pain sensations has recently undergone considerable development.

Another factor that spurred us on to re-examine the problem of pain due to central-nervous-system lesions is the frequent occurrence in patients submitted to thalamic surgery for the treatment of pain syndromes (Cassinari *et al.,* 1963 a and b, 1964; Maspes and Pagni, 1965; Pagni, 1966) of pains different from those that brought them to surgery, the new pains being interpretable as of central origin. One can readily appreciate the dilemma of a surgeon preparing to use stereotactic surgery against one form of pain only to be faced by the possibility that the patient may have to suffer pain even more atrocious than that which brought him to the operating table.

We felt it would then be interesting to make as comprehensive a review as possible of the surgical methods used in the attempt to treat "central pain." It was realized as long ago as the first observations of Déjerine and Roussy (1906) that pains of the central type are usually absolutely refractory to medical treatment. Yet we know of no work in which the results of surgical treatment of central pain have been collected and evaluated.

The physiopathology of central pain has never been thoroughly elucidated. Many theories have been advanced to explain it, and, as we shall see, many of them, especially the earlier ones, were based on theoretical premises that were sometimes flatly contradictory.

At the clinical level the problem is a very complex one. The symptomatology is extremely variable. Even in a single individual various paresthesias may occur in association with excruciating pain and apparently "spontaneous" sensory phenomena in association with phenomena "evoked" by peripheral sensory stimulation. We have asked ourselves whether the injured sensory systems and the physiopathological mechanisms can be the same in cases with pain in the strict sense, in cases with simple paresthesia, in those with "spontaneous" symptoms, and in those with "evoked" phenomena. In the past few workers asked whether the mechanism involved might be different for different symptoms; most centered their attention on pain as such.

Because central sensory phenomena may arise as a result of lesions at any level of the central nervous system, from the spinal cord to the cerebral cortex, the question at once arises whether the pathogenetic mechanism is always the same irrespective of the level involved. Several workers, especially the pioneers in this field, concentrated their attention on the sensation disorders resulting from thalamic lesions and only recently have some tried to answer the broader question.

For our study we have collected from the literature a large number of cases in which subjective sensory phenomena occurred after a surgical lesion of the central nervous system. These phenomena cover an exceedingly wide range of sensations, paresthesias, and pain, mild to extremely violent, spontaneous or evoked. Although at the clinical level subjective manifestations as diverse as these differ radically in importance, for both surgeon and patient, we nonetheless felt that they all could be studied from the same point of view. It is a matter of clinical experience that paresthesias and pains can appear in association in a given individual and that a given anatomicopathological lesion may give rise to simple paresthesia or to excruciating pain.

This vast range of sensations may be termed "subjective sensory phenomena of central origin" (S.S.P.C.O.), both real pain and paresthesia with or without pain being included. Although our approach to the clinical problem of subjective sensory disturbances from central lesions may seem oversimplified, there are two reasons for tackling the problem in this way. First, what we know of the subjective experiences of our patients depends upon their own descriptions. Affect and personality certainly play a major role in each individual's interpretation of his subjective sensory experience. One patient may describe as "troublesome" a paresthesia that another would say was "unbearable." Second, in the literature a given term is used to indicate quite different phenomena and it is therefore sometimes difficult to deduce from the case records the real nature of the disturbances of which the patients complained.

THE PAIN PATHWAYS AND CENTERS

OF THE CENTRAL NERVOUS SYSTEM:

NOTES ON ANATOMY AND PHYSIOLOGY

In this chapter we shall give a schematic exposition of some anatomical and physiological data on the systems of pain transmission, dwelling on some points to which little importance is usually attached but which may be of great interest for the purpose of interpreting central pain.

As is known, the peripheral nerves are made up of several types of fibers, divided into groups according to diameter. There are the A fibers, which may then be divided into subgroups distinguished by the Greek letters: alpha, beta, gamma, delta, and epsilon; and B fibers; and the C fibers. The A fibers are myelinated, the coarsest being 16–20 μ in diameter and the finest 2–4 μ. The C fibers are unmyelinated and are 2 μ or less in diameter. After a great deal of research, it has been concluded that pain sensations are transmitted by the finer A fibers, 2–5 μ in diameter, belonging to the delta and epsilon subgroups and by the unmyelinated C fibers (White and Sweet, 1955).

These A fibers transmit impulses at a high speed, while the finer, unmyelinated fibers transmit them at a lower speed. The two types of fibers are thought to be responsible for two different types of pain sensation: the myelinated fibers of the A delta group are thought to be responsible for clearly localized pain of rapid onset, while the slower-transmitting unmyelinated C fibers mediate poorly localized, dull, aching sensations (White and Sweet, 1955).

The problem of the pathways of pain transmission becomes

more complicated as soon as the fibers enter the spinal cord, for even now there are still many gaps in our knowledge.

Even the way in which the fibers terminate in the spinal cord illustrates the complexity of the problem. The finest fibers of the posterior root, some myelinated but the majority not, come together to form a small bundle situated laterally and enter the tract of Lissauer or fasciculus dorsolateralis. These fibers, which are thought to subserve the transmission of pain sensations, before entering the gray substance of the posterior horns and synapsing with it, divide, like all other sense fibers, into two branches, one ascending and one descending (Ranson and Clark, 1957). Both branches pass into the tract of Lissauer for a short distance only (Pearson, 1952). The fact that the finer fibers, myelinated and unmyelinated, of the posterior roots branch after entering the tract of Lissauer has been known since the time of Ramón y Cajal (1899); see Fig. 1.

Ramón y Cajal (1899) also observed that the unmyelinated fibers, after entering the spinal cord, do not always branch symmetrically Y-fashion and that sometimes one of the branches seems to be a continuation of the main trunk and the other a collateral.

Another very important observation of Ramón y Cajal was that many collaterals ("colaterales") end in the gelatinous substance of Rolando: these various collaterals come both from the tract of Burdach and from the tract of Lissauer ("como de la zona marginal de Lissauer"; Ramón y Cajal, 1899:265).

Sprague and Ha (1964) observed that the finest fibers of the posterior root enter the tract of Lissauer and send collaterals immediately into the gelatinous substance. Szentàgothai (1964) says that the "small-calibered primary sensory fibers (Ranson, 1914, lateral bundle of the dorsal root) . . . may establish synaptic contact with ten neurons" of the gelatinous substance of Rolando.

We feel that these anatomical details are highly relevant to the interpretation of certain central pains due to lesion of the first neuron in the neuraxis, as we shall see later.

Pearson (1952) made a special study of the mode of termination of the fibers of the tract of Lissauer. He observed that "the finely myelinated and unmyelinated dorsal root fibers terminate in the gelatinous substance. Here they can come into synaptic relation with the pericornual cells, the constituent cells of the gelatinous substance, and the dorsal dendrites of the cells of the nucleus proprius. The axons of the cells of the gelatinous substance appear to end in synaptic relation with the pericornual cells and the cells of the nucleus proprius." In particular, "the evidence

FIG. 1. Tangential and longitudinal section of the posterior column, showing bifurcation of fine, unmyelinated C fibers in the tract of Lissauer. Note also that one of the branches seems to be a continuation of the main trunk and the other a collateral. *Source:* Ramón y Cajal (1899).

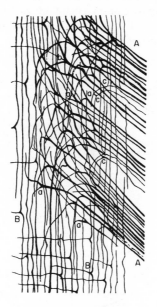

suggests that small . . . fibers relay their impulses through one or more intercalated neurons . . . to the pericornual cells and to cells of the nucleus proprius, which, in turn, give rise to the lateral spinothalamic tract . . . Larger fibers . . . that penetrate or bypass the gelatinous substance also end in synaptic relation to neurons of the nucleus proprius." It must, however, be pointed out that the "fine fibers . . . terminating in a small nodule on a dendrite or on the cell body of a neuron of the nucleus proprius" may give rise during their course through the gelatinous substance of Rolando to a large number of collaterals which end there (Fig. 2). Thus even at the level of the posterior horns of the spinal cord there are thought to be different anatomical substrates for fast pain and for slow pain: the C fibers — at least most of them — transmit their impulses through internuncial neurons of the gelatinous substance, whereas the A fibers

FIG. 2. The A fibers and finer C fibers of the posterior root, before terminating on a dendrite or on a cell body of a neuron of the nucleus proprius, may give rise to collaterals which end in the gelatinous substance of Rolando. *Source:* Pearson (1952).

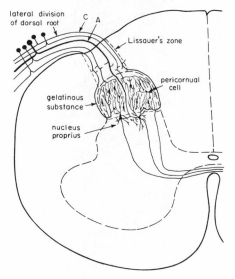

transmit them directly to the cells that give rise to the fibers of the spinothalamic tract (secondary neurons: spinothalamic tract).

White and Sweet (1955) likewise supposed that these two modes of termination might constitute the anatomical basis for the transmission of the two types of pain—fast and slow—identified in peripheral nerves. Further, the mode of termination of the pain-carrying fibers affords ample possibility of interaction and elaboration of the impulses even inside the gelatinous substance, which Bok (1928) regarded as the major associative organ of the posterior horns.

It is important to note that the gelatinous substance and the cells that make it up form a long column extending the whole length of the spinal cord on the tip of the posterior horns and that the gelatinous substance consists largely of small Golgi Type II cells (Ranson and Clark, 1957) whose axons, which are hard to follow through (Pearson, 1952), end in the gelatinous substance itself.

The pericornual and nucleus proprius cells (Fig. 2) give rise to the fibers of the spinothalamic tract, which, after crossing in the anterior commissure, rise along the anterolateral funiculus on the opposite side. It is thought that these fibers are responsible for the transmission of thermal and pain impulses. Actually, the position and degree of crossing of the fibers of the spinothalamic tract vary greatly. It is generally supposed that pain-sense fibers are crossed. But this is not always true: there are cases in which only some of the spinothalamic fibers cross and cases have even been described (Voris, 1957) in which the fibers of the spinothalamic tract get as far as the thalamus without crossing at all and run into the homolateral funiculus.

In reality only a small percentage of these fibers with an ascending course in the anterolateral funiculus, collected in the area that is usually attributed to the spinothalamic tract, reach the relay center of the thalamus. Some time ago Walker (1938, 1940) observed that many fibers of the spinothalamic tract stop at the level of the pons, midbrain, and bulb. This datum has since been confirmed by other workers (Gardner and Cuneo, 1945; Morin *et al.*, 1951; Sie Pek Giok, 1956), who noted that few fibers of the spinothalamic tract actually reach the relay center of the thalamus. Glees and Bailey (1951) and Glees (1953) observed that at the level of the superior colliculus only about 1500–2000 fibers constitute the spinothalamic contingent and reach the thalamus; hence only a few of the fibers really deserve the name of spinothalamic fibers. All the other fibers, which stop at the lower levels of the bulb, pons, and midbrain, are commonly called spinoreticular and spinotectal. It is important to note that, since at spinal level they run mixed with spinothalamic fibers in the strict sense, they are usually included in the "spinothalamic tract" (Noordenbos, 1959).

In the spinal cord of animals and man there are, however, along with the long-fiber systems just mentioned (spinothalamic, spinoreticular, and spinotectal) other systems of neurons and fibers which may take part in the transmission of pain stimuli to the higher centers. These systems, the existence of which has been postulated on anatomicophysiological, experimental, and clinical evidence, would seem to be polysynaptic systems.

In 1895 Fajersztain described this system of polysynaptic fibers as running intimately mixed with fibers of the tracts of long ascending fibers. Goldschneider (1898) and Zihen (1899) accepted the existence of this polysynaptic system in the spinal cord as a pathway of sensory transmission. May (1906) described a short-neuron pathway, which he thought was a secondary pathway for pain impulses to the thalamus: this pathway would, he thought, become usable after lesions of the direct spinothalamic pathway or might have a contributory or replacement function.

Winkler (1917) considered that the fibers of these polysynaptic systems originate in cells of the gelatinous substance or in Gierke's cells and that their course is partly crossed and partly uncrossed. Karplus and Kreidl (1914–1925) and Kletzkin and Spiegel (1952) thought that pain impulses were transmitted even under normal conditions through these short-axon systems of the spinal gray substance.

Certain clinical observations also suggest that there are systems accessory to the spinothalamic tract which subserve the transmission of pain impulses. Rasmussen (1945) and Walker (1940) thought that the pain persisting after cordotomy was due to the coming into operation of these phylogenetically ancient pathways. Osàcar *et al.* (1961), on the strength of a histologically documented case of bilateral section of the anterolateral quadrant of the cord unaccompanied by any alteration of sensibility to temperature and pain, held that a polysynaptic system, which they call the reticular system of the spinal cord, might provide an anatomical basis for the transmission of temperature and pain impulses.

Actually, as Nathan (1956) indicated, there is no absolute anatomical documentation of the site of these short-axon polysynaptic systems: these "short tracts" might be any intrinsic fibers of the posterior columns or of the tract of Lissauer or any fibers of the gray substance. Noordenbos (1959) pointed out that the fibers of this polysynaptic system have been variously named: spinospinal, propriospinal, intrinsic spinal, or fasciculus proprius fibers (Figs. 3–4).

Another point that Ramón y Cajal made long ago is that the fibers of the anterolateral funiculus give rise to numerous collaterals which end by spreading themselves over the gray substance of the cord (Fig. 3).

The long spinothalamic fibers proper end in the specific relay nucleus of the lateral mass of the thalamus. This mass, containing many nuclei, is absent in the lower animals and attains its maximum development in the primates and in man (Brower, 1933). The exact mode of termination of the spinothalamic fibers is still a matter of debate, though all are agreed that they

FIG. 3. Diagram of the ascending systems subserving the transmission of pain stimuli.

(a) True spinothalamocortical fibers. The spinothalamic fibers originating in the nucleus proprius and pericornual cells of the posterior horns reach the thalamus, where they end in the VPL relay nucleus, though some of them reach the CM and other nuclei of the diffuse projection system. From these fibers stem collaterals bound for the gray substance of the spinal cord and the reticular systems of the brainstem. (b) Long spinospinal fibers (which arise and end in the gray substance of the spinal cord), spinoreticular fibers (which are bound for the reticular formations of the bulb, pons, and midbrain), and spinotectal fibers. These long fibers run united with the spinothalamic fibers proper in the anterolateral funiculus of the cord in the area marked "spinothalamic tract": they branch off at various levels from the spinothalamic fibers proper. (c) System of short-axon neurons which constitute the "polysynaptic system" of the spinal cord, which reaches the thalamus via the reticular formations of the brainstem. Onto this system converge the collaterals of (a) and the fibers of (b). (d) Nucleus centrum medianum (CM) and internal medullary lamina region. (e) Nuclei VPL and VPM.

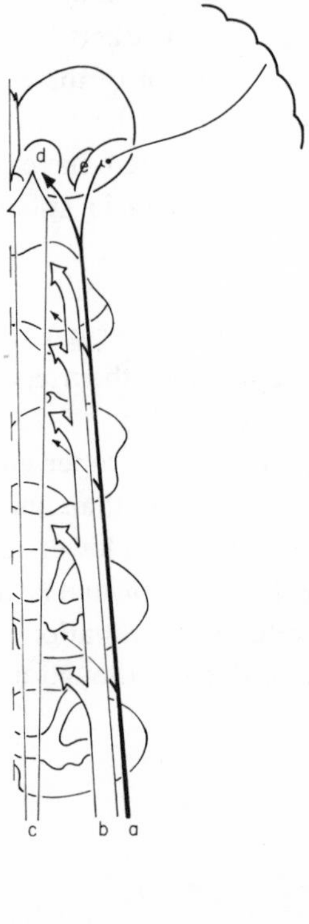

end in the inferolateral posterior portion of the lateral mass of the thalamus in the region that American workers call the ventro-postero-lateral and ventro-postero-medial nuclei, where the medial lemniscus and quintothalamic tract fibers end also. Some (Bailey *et al.*, 1954; Glees, 1961) considered that the fibers of the medial lemniscus and of the spinothalamic tract at the level of the posterior ventral nucleus are superposed or partly so, and hence their impulses end on groups of intermixed cells or might even converge on the same cell. Other workers maintain that there is a specific region in which the spinothalamic fibers end. As early as 1938 Walker observed that in chimpanzees the fibers of the spinothalamic tract end in the posterior basal portion of the lateral mass of the thalamus and those of the medial lemniscus in front of the spinothalamic fibers. Hassler (1960) thought that the spinothalamic tract ended in a very restricted area of the posterolateral nucleus, which he identified as the more basal portion of this nucleus and which he called the "parvicellular caudal ventral nucleus" on account of the size of the cells constituting it. Hassler's view, based on the results of anatomical studies in man and on some comparative anatomy data (Mehler, 1957), appears

FIG. 4. Diagram showing the distribution of the intrinsic fibers of the spinal cord in the monkey. This diagram shows only the fibers of the white substance and not the propriospinal fibers of the gray substance, which may constitute a large part of the "polysynaptic systems" of the spinal cord, according to Nathan (1956). *Source:* Tower, *et al.* (1941).

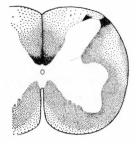

to be confirmed by the stereotactic surgery experience of Hassler and Riechert (1959).

Within the posterior ventral nuclei there is a somatotopic representation of the various districts of the body, although there is much overlapping. There is also thought to be some slight degree of bilateral representation. Bowsher (1957) observed, when studying the operative specimens of cordotomized patients, that the spinothalamic tract fibers ended in the homolateral and contralateral posterolateral ventral nuclei; before reaching the contralateral thalamus the fibers cross in the dorsal part of the posterior commissure. It would therefore seem to be demonstrated that even at thalamic level there is bilateral representation of pain sensation.

The existence of fibers of the anterolateral funiculus of the spinal cord running united with the spinothalamic fibers and ending in the reticular formations of the brainstem is, as we said earlier, now documented by extensive literature on animals (Johnson, 1954; Rossi and Brodal, 1957; Mehler *et al.,* 1956) and on man (Bowsher, 1957, 1959, 1960). See Fig. 5. We have also pointed out that only the fibers that reach the thalamus and end in its relay nuclei deserve the name of spinothalamic fibers proper. Not even all the fibers that reach the thalamus end in the specific sensory relay nuclei. In 1938 Walker noted that in chimpanzees a number of spinothalamic tract fibers end outside the lateral mass of the thalamus "in the nuclei of the midline of the thalamus." Bowsher (1957) stated categorically that in man the fibers of the spinothalamic tract may end in the reticular nucleus of the thalamus and in the center median nucleus. He emphasized the point that although it had been observed in the past that the spinothalamic tract fibers cross the center median nucleus no one had ever proved that some of them could end there (Figs. 4–5). According to Hassler (1960), many fibers of the spinothalamic system stop in the nuclei of the diffuse projection system of the thalamus (nuclei of the lamina medullaris thalami,

14

nucleus limitans); nevertheless, he denied that the uncrossed fibers reach the center median nucleus directly, although he admitted that impulses might reach it through the reticular formation of the brainstem. Moreover, he was convinced that the brainstem and the thalamic diffuse projection system send their fibers to the caudate nucleus, putamen, and globus pallidus.

Full accordance is not yet reached on whether the nucleus centrum medianum is or is not a significant neural relay in the central pain pathway. Mehler (1966) suggests that pain mechanisms might be represented by lower neural structures in mesencephalon or in the region of the mesodiencephalic transition.

FIG. 5. Diagram of the termination of the spinoreticular fibers in the reticular formations of the brainstem.
(1) Tractus spinothalamicus; (2) obex; (3) formatio reticularis medullae oblongatae; (4) nucleus gigantocellularis; (5) ventriculus quartus; (6) formatio reticularis pontis; (7) tegmentum and tectum mesencephali; (8) centrum medianum thalami; (9) nucleus posterolateralis thalami; (10) nucleus reticularis thalami; (11) commissura posterior. *Source:* D. Bowsher (1957).

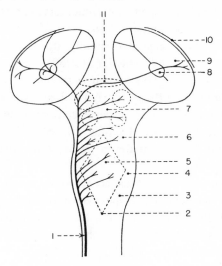

Notwithstanding these discrepancies, it is thus anatomically documented that some fibers of the so-called spinothalamic tract actually end in the reticular formations of the brainstem and in the thalamic diffuse projection system. There is a vast mass of anatomicophysiological data (Macchi and Angeleri, 1957; Rossi and Zanchetti, 1957) demonstrating the intimate connections between the reticular formations of the bulb, pons, and mid-brain, and the formations of the thalamic diffuse projection system.

There is a tendency to assign to these reticular systems, which are thought to take part in the regulation of a large number of central nervous system functions, a fundamental role in the process of transmission and perception of pain stimuli. The perception of certain pain sensations might occur at subcortical level within these systems, which do not belong to the specific system represented by the spinothalamocortical pathway. This opinion is based on the observation that the lower animals, in which the cortex and the neothalamus with the specific nuclei—usually regarded as mediating the transmission of pain impulses in man—are either absent or rudimentary, can still experience pain (Brower, 1933; Mehler, 1966).

Bowsher (1957) suggested calling this the "spinoreticulo-thalamic system" and Hassler (1960) suggested "trunko-thalamische System." This system is thought to have the property of transmitting diffuse, poorly localized pain sensations that last for a long time and are experienced for some time after the stimulus. The nature of the pain transmitted by this system would be easy to account for in terms of its anatomicophysiological characteristics.

These concepts have been accepted by many workers concerned with the treatment of pain by stereotactic surgery (Mark et al., 1960; Bettag and Yoshida, 1960; Cassinari et al., 1964), and they seem to be supported by the clinical results as well as by the anatomical evidence (Mark et al., 1963).

This enormously complex organization of the pathways of pain transmission is shown schematically in Fig. 3, in which the spinothalamic pathway proper, originating in the cells of the nucleus proprius or in the pericornual cells of the posterior horns, is shown as a continuous line rising from the spinal cord to the posterior ventral nucleus of the thalamus (Fig. 3a). The polysynaptic system (Fig. 3c) is represented by an arrow rising from the lower spinal cord to the center median nucleus. Long fibers, running for some distance united to the spinothalamic tract and leaving it to end in the polysynaptic system at various levels, are represented by other arrows (Fig. 3b); these long fibers may be considered as belonging to the spinoreticulothalamic system. It should also be noted that the spinothalamic fibers send many collaterals to the spinoreticulothalamic system.

One peculiar aspect of the anatomical organization of the pain pathways concerns the trigeminal system. It is now universally accepted that the most caudal part of the nucleus of the descending tract of the trigeminal nerve (nucleus tractus spinalis trigemini caudalis of Olszewski, 1950) transmits pain and temperature sensations.

An important anatomical feature of the caudal nucleus of V is that it also receives impulses from other nerves (VII, IX, and X), from the contralateral homologous nucleus, and from the cuneate nuclei. The posterior root fibers, after entering the pons, bend caudal to reach the nucleus caudalis. Many of them do not branch, but some divide into two branches: one ascending and the other descending. The descending branches, after giving off many collaterals ("la rama descendente . . . emite en su curso infinidad de colaterales"—Ramón y Cajal, 1899; Brodal, 1950) —which end in the descending nucleus and probably even in the bulbar reticular substance—end in the nucleus caudalis and synapse with the quintothalamic neurons. The exact anatomical sites of the secondary neurons originating in the nucleus caudalis are still unknown. According to Stewart and King (1961, 1963; Stewart et al., 1963, 1964), who have made a thorough histologic and physiological study of the connections of this nucleus in cats, it is possible to distinguish three ascending pathways from the nucleus: (a) a fast pathway with a bilateral distribution, the neurons of which end in the nucleus arcuatus of the ventrobasal complex of the thalamus (i.e., VPM in man)—quintothalamic neurons—and in the intralaminar-center median nucleus system of the thalamus; they emphasize the fact that only the caudal portion of the descending nucleus of the trigeminal has direct connections with the intralaminar-center median nucleus system of the thalamus; (b) a polysynaptic pathway with a diffuse bilateral distribution to the reticular formations of the midbrain, to the magnocellular portion of the geniculate body, and to certain hypothalamo-diencephalic regions; (c) an "intranuclear" pathway ascending to the trigeminal nucleus and terminating in the reticular formations of the bulb, pons, and midbrain and in the more cranial portion of the sensory nucleus of the trigeminal nerve.

The hypothesis of thalamoparietal fibers specifically subserving the transmission of pain impulses and of a cortical area specifically subserving the reception of pain impulses is accepted by many workers but rejected by others. There is certainly scant anatomical or physiological evidence either for the fibers or for the area. Indeed, in 1962 Bishop stated that the only pathway that can be regarded as having a projection to a specific area of the cortex is the medial lemniscus.

In this connection White and Sweet (1955) said: "It is pertinent to point out that we do not know what fibers or tract may be specifically concerned with the transmission of pain impulses beyond the termination of the secondary afferent neurons wherever they may happen to end in the spinal cord, brainstem or thalamus."

Biemond (1956) pointed out that up to 1956 very little was known for sure about the cortical projection of pain and it was commonly thought that the pain fibers at suprathalamic level mix diffusely with the other sensory fibers to reach the postcentral gyrus. However, on the strength of certain anatomical and clinical observations Biemond thought it safe to say that there is a specific area of the cortex to which pain fibers project: this area is thought to be the second sensory area of Penfield, which lies on the upper lip of the fissure of Sylvius.

Hassler (1960), on the other hand, also on the strength of anatomical findings in man, stated that the parvicellular ventrocaudal nucleus, which he regards as the point of arrival of the spinothalamic fibers, projects to area 3B of the postcentral cortex. He reported on the results of physiological studies by Melzack and Haugen (1957) which are said to demonstrate a special projection of the pain fibers to the postcentral cortex as well as to the second somatic area. Mountcastle and Powell (1959) demonstrated in the postcentral gyrus of monkeys, cellular elements that are activated by nociceptive cutaneous stimuli. Carreras and Visintini (1965) made similar observations in the cat. Ranson and Clark (1957) held that there is cortical projection of pain sensation to the postcentral gyrus.

Hassler (1960) considered, however, that the cortical representations are of less importance than the thalamic representations for the appreciation of pain. Bowsher (1957) was of the same opinion. According to him, if there is cortical representation of pain it must be very minor, given the small number of spinothalamic pain fibers reaching the posterior ventral nucleus of the thalamus.

In support of the view that there is a parietal localization of pain there are many clinical and anatomicoclinical observations of localized parietal lesions, without involvement of the thalamus, in which clinical examination disclosed derangement of the pain sense (analgesia or hypoalgesia) and in some cases central pain (Guillain and Bertrand, 1932; Davison and Schick, 1935; Lhermitte and Ajuraguerra, 1935; Marshall, 1951; Façon et al., 1960). Talairach et al. (1960) made a careful review of the literature on this subject.

In short, many workers consider that the parietal cortex plays a direct part in the elaboration of pain sensations (Marshall,

1951; Hoff *et al.,* 1953; Biemond, 1956; Façon *et al.,* 1960) whereas others consider that the conscious integration of these sensations occurs mainly, if not solely, at subcortical level (Head and Holmes, 1911; Ajuraguerra, 1937; Walker, 1938; Guillaume and Sigwald, 1947; Wycis and Spiegel, 1962). Even cortical stimulation experiments in man have failed to provide a final answer on this point. Penfield and Boldrey (1937) elicited a definite pain sensation in only 11 out of 426 stimulations of the parietal cortex; in the majority of cases there were sensations of various kinds but not pain. Jung (1959) went so far as to say that cortical stimulation in man never causes pain and that in the rare instances in which it has been observed it was really due to stimulation of the walls of blood vessels. Further, if the second somatic area were specifically concerned with the reception of pain stimuli, as Biemond (1956) would have us believe, stimulation of it should give rise mainly to pain sensations. Yet, according to the experiments of Penfield and Jasper (1954), the sensations evoked by stimulating this region do not differ in the main from those aroused by stimulating the postcentral cortex. In any case, Hécaen *et al.* (1949) reported that they had found an area in the white substance of the parietal lobe about 2.5 cm from the supralateral surface, deep-lying, in which mild electrical stimuli gave rise to violent, localized shooting pains. These data would appear to prove the existence of fibers specifically concerned with the transmission of pain in the subcortical white substance.

In the anatomical organization of the temperature and pain sense systems it must not be forgotten that there are corticofugal fibers bound not only for the thalamic nuclei but also for the subthalamic relay stations (Walker, 1938; Foerster, 1927; Walshe, 1959).

The organization of the thalamopetal fibers is roughly superposable on that of the thalamofugal systems (Walker, 1938). Head and Holmes (1911) thought that these fibers exerted an inhibitory action on the thalamus. The action of these corticofugal systems is most probably very complex: they are thought to exert a regulating action upon the activity of the thalamic nuclei and of the subthalamic relay stations and upon the transmission of afferent impulses to the cortex (Brower, 1933; Gobbel and Liles, 1945; Fulton, 1951; Haghbarth and Kerr, 1954; Livingston, 1959).

At this point it might be well to schematize the salient data that have emerged from this brief survey of current thinking on the anatomical organization of the pain pathways. There are two systems concerned with the transmission of pain impulses:

Paucisynaptic System (*Spinothalamocortical*). This is a phylogenetically recent pathway consisting of only three neurons: the *first neuron,* originating in the cells of the spinal ganglia and of the gasserian ganglion, enters the neuraxis and ends, directly or indirectly, on the *second neuron,* which lies in the posterior horns of the spinal cord (pericornual cell and nucleus proprius cell) or in the gelatinous nucleus of the spinal tract of the trigeminal nerve, from which the spinothalamic and quintothalamic fibers originate; they in their turn end on the *third neuron,* which lies in the posterior ventral nuclei of the thalamus and projects, via the thalamocortical fibers, to the sensory cortex. The organization of this system is relatively simple and interruption of the transmission of pain impulses along it is relatively easy, although the collaterals of these fibers bound for the reticular formations may divert the impulses to other systems.

Polysynaptic System (*Spinoreticulothalamic*). This is a phylogenetically old pathway with a complex anatomical constitution within which pain impulses are possibly transmitted to the higher centers via chains of short-axon neurons. To this system, which extends from the spinal cord to the thalamus and which is called the spinoreticulothalamic system, belong the propriospinal systems, the reticular systems of the brainstem and thalamus, the so-called spinoreticular fibers. Moreover, at any level of the neuraxis pain impulses converge on this system via the collaterals of the fibers of the paucisynaptic system.

This system is probably of fundamental importance in the transmission of pain impulses even in health and perhaps predominates after lesions to the paucisynaptic system. It must be

FIG. 6. Diagram of surgical operations on the neuraxis that have given rise to central pain. At whatever level of the second and third neurons the paucisynaptic pathway is interrupted, pain impulses can always be diverted and conveyed by the polysynaptic systems. The higher the level of interruption of the spinothalamic tract, the greater the number of fibers that can convey pain impulses in the polysynaptic systems. See Fig. 3 for further explanations.

(a) True spinothalamic fibers; (b) spinospinal, spinoreticular, and spinotectal long fibers; (c) polysynaptic systems of the spinal cord and brainstem; (1) dorsal spinothalamic tractotomy; (2) cervical spinothalamic tractotomy; (3) spinothalamic tractotomy at bulbar level; (4) spinothalamic tractotomy at mesencephalic level; (5) stereotactic operation: thalamotomy of the VPM-VPL nuclei.

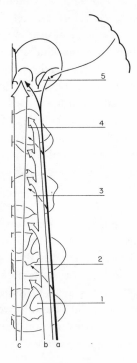

remembered that at whatever level of the neuraxis interruption of the paucisynaptic system occurs the pain impulses can be switched to the polysynaptic system. Although this is readily understandable (Fig. 6) for lesions of the second and third neuron of the paucisynaptic pathway, it may not seem to fit lesions affecting the first neuron in the neuraxis. Yet, in this type of lesion also pain impulses can be switched to the polysynaptic systems.

Indeed, as soon as the A fibers have entered the tract of Lis-

FIG. 7. Diagram illustrating the mode of termination of the A and C fibers (primary neurons) in the spinal cord. Both the A and C fibers bifurcate into an ascending and a descending branch and throw off collaterals which end in the gelatinous substance of Rolando. Through these collaterals impulses may reach the cells of the gelatinous substance, which probably belong to the polysynaptic system of the spinal cord. The ascending branches of the A fibers end on the cells that give rise to the spinothalamic fibers proper (secondary neurons of the paucisynaptic pathway). If a lesion interrupts fiber A before it synapses with the second neuron, pain impulses may be switched onto the polysynaptic system and be conveyed along it to higher levels.
(a) A and C fibers. (b) The arrow "b" represents the polysynaptic ascending system of the gelatinous substance of Rolando.

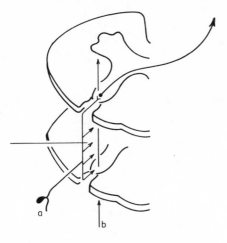

FIG. 8. Summary diagram of the trigeminal sensory pathway and of the mode of termination of the pain fibers of V. The pain fibers descend as far as the "subnucleus gelatinosus," where they synapse with the cells of origin of the quintothalamic tract (second neuron of the paucisynaptic pathway). These descending fibers—many of which do not bifurcate though some give rise to an ascending branch—throw off numerous collaterals. A lesion of the descending fibers leaves intact the ascending branches of the bifurcating fibers and all the collaterals originating above the lesion. Pain impulses are probably diverted via the spared collaterals onto the polysynaptic systems of the brainstem and of the "intranuclear pathway" and thence conveyed to higher levels.

(a) Nucleus oralis; (b) nucleus interpolaris; (c) nucleus caudalis, which receives all the pain fibers of V; (d) cervical region where the nucleus caudalis continues with the gelatinous substance of Rolando; (e) posterior cervical root; (f) spinothalamic tract; (g) quintothalamic tract; (h) sensory root of the trigeminal nerve; (i) "intranuclear pathway" (polysynaptic), which transmits impulses to the reticular formations of the brainstem; (r) reticular formations of the brainstem; (l) surgical section of the descending trigeminal root at obex level, which may involve the trigeminal sensory nucleus at a deep level.

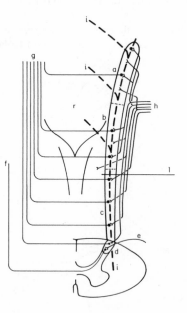

sauer they bifurcate, forming an ascending and a descending branch. The ascending branch reaches the second neuron of the paucisynaptic pathway. The collaterals of the ascending and descending branches and the descending branch itself can end in the gelatinous substance of Rolando.

The C fibers likewise divide into two branches, which only occasionally end on the second neuron of the spinothalamic paucisynaptic pathway (Pearson, 1952). They are usually bound for the small cells of the gelatinous substance and their impulses are transmitted through the numerous intercalary neurons of that substance.

Hence, interruption of the first neuron immediately after its entry into the neuraxis above the point of entry of a root will enable the impulses to escape through the descending branch or the spared collaterals. Even if these impulses do not reach the cells of origin of the spinothalamic fibers (second neuron) they can still reach other neurons, that is, the small cells of the gelatinous substance, which probably belong to the polysynaptic system (Fig. 7). It is likely that a similar mechanism operates at the bulbar level following interruption of the descending root of the trigeminal; when the fibers carrying the pain impulses are interrupted before their entry into the "gelatinous substance of the spinal tract" (subnucleus gelatinosus), which is the homolog of the gelatinous substance of Rolando in the spinal cord, it is probable that even though the impulses can no longer reach the cells of origin of the quintothalamic tract they are diverted through collaterals in front of the lesion to other pathways (Fig. 8).

It is well known from the meticulous research of Windle (1926) that, if there are definitely trigeminal fibers which after entering the pons descend without bifurcating into the descending root of V, "some of the fibers of fine caliber bifurcate in the same way as the heavy ones" and that "some fibers, not all coarse . . . give off an extremely delicate branch that . . . often apparently ends in that region of transition between the 'main sensory nucleus' and the 'nucleus of the spinal tract.' "

PATHOLOGICAL ANATOMY

OF SPONTANEOUS LESIONS

CAUSING CENTRAL PAIN

The lesions responsible for central pain and related phenomena may be vascular lesions of the ischemic or hemorrhagic type (Ajuraguerra, 1937; Garcin, 1937; Riddoch, 1938), expanding lesions (Ajuraguerra, 1937; Garcin, 1937; Riddoch, 1938; Smyth and Stern, 1938; Clarke, 1898; Hyndman and van Hepps, 1939; Amici, 1955; Tovi *et al.,* 1961), traumatic and degenerative lesions (Garcin, 1937; Ajuraguerra, 1937; Riddoch, 1938). Central pain may be caused by lesions at any level of the neuraxis. The lesions we have mentioned are observed with varying frequency at different levels of the central nervous system; this explains why the type of lesion most often blamed for the onset of central pain varies according to the region of the neuraxis considered. In the literature, for example, it is sometimes stated that in the majority of cases the cause of pains of thalamic origin is a vascular lesion of the ischemic type, although vascular lesions do not generally seem to be the cause of pains of spinal origin. Actually, according to recent statistics, tumors of the thalamus often do give rise to subjective sensory phenomena with pain (Tovi *et al.,* 1961; Amici, 1955). Expanding lesions, especially tuberculomas, are regarded as the most frequent cause of pain in lesions of the pons.

In the following review of the literature our main purpose will be to establish which system(s) of fibers or cells were affected at the various levels of the neuraxis in cases in which subjective central phenomena occurred. There are many reports in the literature on this subject, most of them old. As we shall see, the conclusions of the various workers who have tried on the basis of this material to identify the structure in which lesions are responsible for the onset of central pain sometimes conflict. The divergence of opinion is fairly easily explained by the fact that spontaneous lesions are usually extensive, difficult to define, often plurifocal, and affect several systems with different functions.

We will now briefly review the salient data of the literature on the subject.

SPINAL CORD

According to Garcin (1937), the spinal cord lesions that can give rise to central pain are (a) wounds and injuries; (b) intramedullary lesions; (c) syringomyelia; (d) disseminated sclerosis and amyotrophic lateral sclerosis; and (e) vascular lesions of the cord.

The structures of the cord in which lesions may cause pain of the central type are (1) cells of the posterior horns; (2) the spinothalamic tract; (3) sensory pathways of the posterior funiculi (Garcin, 1937; Riddoch, 1938). According to Lhermitte (1933), on the other hand, pains from spinal lesions are not due to involvement of the spinothalamic pathway transmitting pain but to lesions of the dorsal part of the spinal cord, that is of the posterior funiculi.

All workers are agreed that when central pain arises as a result of cord lesions there is always lesion of sensory structures, whether they be cells or fibers mediating pain stimuli (spinothalamic pathway) or cells or fibers mediating the stimuli of epicritic sensibility (posterior funiculi).

BULB AND PONS

The bulbar lesions occasioning central pain are generally ischemic vascular lesions from occlusion of the inferior posterior cerebellar artery, which causes a lesion of the spinothalamic pathway and of the nucleus and/or of the descending root of the trigeminal nerve on the same side, which at clinical level means an alternating sensory syndrome (Wallenberg's syndrome).

Lesions of the pons, on the other hand, are often due to tuberculomas, but even at this level the sensory structures may be affected (Ajuraguerra, 1937). In these cases there may also be involvement of Reil's band (medial lemniscus) and of the reticular formations (Ajuraguerra, 1937).

Most bulbopontine lesions with central pain are accompanied by altered sensibility to temperature and pain on the contralateral half of the body due to lesion of the spinothalamic tract. In some cases loss of sensibility to temperature and pain is accompanied by loss of epicritic sensibility due to extension of the lesion to Reil's band. There are, however, extremely rare cases in the literature in which it would seem that a central pain was present without the possibility of demonstrating any temperature-pain sense deficit, there being loss of epicritic sensibility only. At least at the clinical level, involvement of the spinothalamic tract must be ruled out in these cases. Ajuraguerra in his monograph (1937) reports three cases in which central pain was unaccompanied by any sensory deficit; in these cases one can only presume that both the spinothalamic tract and Reil's band were spared.

Although the anatomical evidence shows that most cases of bulbopontine pain are due to lesions involving the spinothalamic paucisynaptic pathway of pain transmission, either alone or in association with the pathways of epicritic sensibility, there would appear to be cases of bulbopontine central pain with lesion of Reil's band only (Garcin, 1937) or even cases in which the long pathways of sensibility are spared. Two cases reported by Ajuraguerra (1937) are of particular interest in this connection: in both cases the sensory pathways were intact and in one it seems that there was an "atteinte isolée de la substance réticulée."

MIDBRAIN

Garcin (1937) reported no cases of central pain due to mid-brain lesions. Riddoch (1938) claimed that this was due to the lack of gray sensory nuclei in the midbrain. Noordenbos (1959) pointed out that central pain from spontaneous midbrain lesions is very rare but that pain due to surgical lesions of the spino-thalamic tract at mesencephalic level is very common.

THALAMUS

Thalamic lesions often cause central pain. Generally, tha-lamic pain is due to vascular, ischemic, or hemorrhagic lesions. Not all thalamic lesions cause pain, and this is why many workers in the past sought to identify the thalamic nuclei that must be injured for pain to arise. Head and Holmes (1911) blamed the lateral area of the thalamus, the point of arrival of the corticothalamic fibers with an inhibitory function. Later, Sager blamed the lateral nucleus of the thalamus, which in von Monakow's classification corresponds to the dorsal part of the external nucleus.

In 1937 Ajuraguerra reviewed all the anatomicoclinical cases of thalamic pain. On the basis of this material and a number of personal cases, he formulated the following hypothesis: with rare exceptions thalamic syndromes with pain are due to a lesion of the "lateral" nucleus of the thalamus or the dorsal part of the external nucleus of von Monakow's classification, von Mona-kow's "lateral" nucleus corresponding to the lateral posterior and lateral dorsal (LP and LD) nuclei of Walker's classification (1938). These nuclei are associative nuclei which receive fibers from the lateral ventral nuclei and from other thalamic nuclei and send fibers to the parietal lobe, with the exception of the postcentral gyrus (Starzl and Magoun, 1951; Peele, 1954). Ajuraguerra and Hécaen (1954) stated that the posterior portion of the "lateral" nucleus, which is supplied by the lenticulo-optic artery and which corresponds to the upper half of the external nucleus of von Monakow and of Foix and Nicolesco, entered into a relation with the parietal lobe "à l'exclusion de la circonvolution pariétale ascendante."

According to Ajuraguerra (1937), although the thalamic pain syndrome is generally due to an ischemic lesion in the territory of the thalamogeniculate artery—which, of course, also supplies the ventral part of the external nucleus of von Monakow's classification, the arrival point of the sensory fibers—it is manifested only when the softening extends upward and involves the superior portion of the external nucleus, that is, von Monakow's "lateral" nucleus. If the lesion is confined to the ventral part of the external nucleus, the arrival point of the sensory fibers, it gives rise to the "analgic" form of the thalamic syndrome, marked by derangement of sensibility without central pain. In support of these assertions Ajuraguerra reported that there are also "hemialgic" forms of the thalamic syndromes, that is, cases in which the thalamic lesion causes central pain and related phenomena without objective derangement of sensibility. These "hemialgic" forms are likewise exceptional and are thought to be due to an ischemic lesion in the territory of the lenticulo-optic arteries supplying the dorsal portion of the external nucleus of the thalamus, that is, von Monakow's "lateral" nucleus. Ajuraguerra himself recognized that these "hemialgic" forms are exceptional; he had found only two cases in the literature. In short, if we have not misunderstood Ajuraguerra's view, the onset of pain due to a thalamic lesion has nothing to do with lesions of the sensory relay nuclei of the thalamus.

Walker (1938) took the opposite view. According to him lesions that give rise to spontaneous pains and to thalamic hyperpathia affect the part of the thalamus in which the somatic sensory systems terminate. His conclusions coincide perfectly with those of Schuster (1936) and, like him, Walker did not rule out the possibility that lesions of the medial nuclei of the thalamus might have something to do with the pathogenesis of these disorders. A case of craniofacial pain recently reported by Rowbotham (1960) is interesting in this connection: in this case histopathologic examination disclosed cellular alterations of the center median and posterior ventral nuclei on both sides.

Ajuraguerra (1937) himself had observed painless cases of lesion of the "lateral" nuclei of the thalamus according to von Monakow's classification. To explain this apparent contradiction with his anatomicoclinical deductions he stated that the nature of the lesion might be of some importance in the pathogenesis of central pain, as well as "individual variations" (unspecified).

The pathological anatomy of spontaneous thalamic lesions accompanied by central pain supplies other evidence in support of Walker's as against Ajuraguerra's hypothesis.

Hoffmann (1933) reported a case of thalamic syndrome caused by a tiny lesion in the most basal part of the posterolateral ventral nucleus. According to Hassler (1960) this was the smallest lesion reported in the literature to be accompanied by a thalamic pain syndrome and must have been located in the basal portion of the VPL nucleus in which, according to him, the spinothalamic fibers arrive and which in his classification is called the ventro-caudal-parvicellular nucleus.

Garcin and Lapresle (1954) reported a case of thalamic pain with a chiro-oral distribution; histopathologic examination revealed a small lesion confined to the inferior internal part of the VPL nucleus and to the more external part of the VPM nucleus.

These observations, especially that of Garcin and Lapresle (1954), which clearly documents the existence of thalamic pain syndromes with a segmental distribution, are in our opinion evidence for Walker's hypothesis as opposed to that of Ajuraguerra. It must be pointed out that Ajuraguerra was unable to supply evidence for the existence of a somatotopic representation in the "lateral" nucleus (von Monakow's classification).

It has been stated repeatedly in the literature that thalamic tumors rarely cause central pain (Imber, 1930; Ajuraguerra,

1937; Garcin, 1937). Yet there are data, especially in the recent literature, which testify to the contrary (Tovi *et al.,* 1961; Amici, 1955). It seems that even in cases of thalamic tumor, involvement of the relay nuclei is of fundamental importance in the genesis of central pain. Smyth and Stern (1938) stated that tumors that invade the thalamus from the ventrolateral side frequently give rise to central pain, whereas those arising within the thalamus and not destroying the ventrolateral part of the thalamus or involving it only secondarily, give rise less often to central pain.

CEREBRAL CORTEX AND SUBCORTICAL REGION

It appears certain that a central pain syndrome can arise as the result of cortico-subcortical lesions that at least macroscopically spare the optic thalamus (Garcin, 1937; Ajuraguerra, 1937; Riddoch, 1938). Talairach *et al.* (1960) recently examined the literature on the subject. The lesions in question are space-occupying lesions, vascular lesions, and traumatic lesions. Some workers include under the heading of cortical central pain that of certain convulsive seizures (Ajuraguerra, 1937; Riddoch, 1938). Garcin (1937), however, considered that the diffusion of the epileptic stimulus to the thalamic nuclei plays a part in the causation of these pains.

As far as we know, central pains due to cortical lesions have been described only in connection with lesions of the parietal regions, especially of the ascending parietal region. Biemond (1956) reported a case of a cortical lesion in a region corresponding roughly to somatic area S II, with pains of the central type.

It is emphasized, however, that in these cases there may be retrograde degenerative lesions of the cells of the thalamic nuclei and that these may be the true cause of pain from parietal lesions.

NONSENSORY STRUCTURES

In the literature there are descriptions of cases of central pains due to lesions of the lenticular nucleus, of the caudate nucleus, and of the infundibulum. Foerster considered that these pains were due to a release of the thalamus from the inhibitory influence that the striated structures are thought to exert over it. Garcin (1937) thought that in these cases pain was really due to involvement of the nearby optic thalamus.

Discussion

From the anatomicopathological evidence of cases of pain syndromes due to spontaneous lesions of the central nervous system we do not feel that any final conclusion can be drawn regarding the structures that must be injured before a pain syndrome can arise. As we have seen, diametrically opposed conclusions have been reached on this point. If a lesion of the sensory pathways and systems would seem to be necessary in the majority of cases, as some workers maintain, it would also seem that central pain is possible without lesion of these systems. This thesis would seem to be supported by Ajuraguerra's cases of pure "hemialgic" thalamic syndromes in which pain was not accompanied by any objective derangement of sensibility.

Only a few workers have asked whether a lesion of the pathways of pain transmission is strictly necessary or whether a lesion of the pathways of epicritic sensibility is sufficient to cause pain. We feel that no answer can be given to the latter question on the basis of the evidence so far considered, because of the massive and extensive nature of the lesions studied. In our view these doubts and problems can be tackled more effectively by studying cases of pain and related sensory phenomena resulting from surgical lesions of the nervous system, and it is with these that we shall deal in the next chapter.

SURGICAL OPERATIONS ON

THE NEURAXIS THAT HAVE GIVEN RISE

TO CENTRAL PAIN

A dreaded risk of operations designed to relieve pain is the possible onset of central pain. Though rare in some types of operations, this complication occurs very frequently in others.

Surgical lesions are usually small and carefully centered on chosen structures; hence the study of the results is almost on a par with experimental research. We therefore feel that a detailed study of the cases in the literature in which the onset of pain and related phenomena were observed might help to solve the problem of the physiopathogenesis of central pain because we know more precisely the site of the lesion in these cases.

We shall give as detailed a review as possible of the case material in the literature we have been able to consult directly. Our review is naturally incomplete, especially with regard to the commoner operations on which there is a vast amount of literature. On anterolateral cordotomy we have consulted only the more recent references; for other operations—mesencephalotomy and stereotactic procedures—the review is more complete.

We have not confined ourselves simply to collecting the data for the surgery of pain but we have also collected as many as possible of the data relating to operations performed for other reasons (extrapyramidal syndromes, encephalopathy of children, spastic syndromes) which might involve a lesion of the pathways of pain or of epicritic sensibility. Probably, however, the workers handling the latter operations, being concerned with other problems, did not devote much attention to the problems of central sensory phenomena. For these reasons it is not possible to attribute a strictly statistical significance to the following data, but we think they are significant for our purpose.

ANTEROLATERAL CORDOTOMY (FIG. 9)

Babtchine (1936), commenting on 47 cases of cordotomy, pointed out that sometimes relapsing pain may be due to "thalamic" central mechanisms, though he did not specify which; these are thus not true relapses but pains which the author thought were probably of central origin.

Dogliotti (1937) stated that after anterolateral cordotomy central pains can arise even when the pain pathways have been completely interrupted.

Sasaki (1938) observed postoperative paresthesia in seven out of 19 cases.

Guillaume and Mazars (1949) reported no paresthesias or central pains in a series of 26 cases treated with cervical cordotomy.

Siöqvist (1950) performed 71 operations on 58 patients: five patients complained of an unpleasant sensation of heat or cold in

FIG. 9. Diagram of an anterolateral cordotomy. This operation interrupts both the spinothalamic fibers proper and other systems of ascending fibers concerned with the transmission of pain stimuli (spinoreticular, spinotectal, and propriospinal fibers of the white substance and of the gray substance).

(1) Lateral pyramidal tract; (2) spinothalamic tract; (3) extrapyramidal pathways; (4) anterior pyramidal tract.

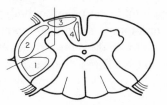

the hypoalgesic area; six others complained of burning pains in that area.

Miserocchi (1951) pointed out that the onset of paresthesias after cordotomy can make the result less satisfactory. He considered that these paresthesias may be due to the lesion of other systems of fibers in the anterolateral funiculus of the cord not essentially concerned with sensibility to temperature and pain. He noted also that the raising of the body temperature sometimes brings on "troublesome" paresthesias in the thermo-analgesic territories but that these disappear with normalization of body temperature.

Lapresle and Guiot (1953) performed anterolateral cordotomy on eight patients suffering from chronic arthrosis of the hip joint. The primary pains disappeared in all cases, but in five cases there appeared an entirely new kind of pain which the patients said was quite different from the pain of their original disease. The new pains appeared within a few days to a few months after operation, usually a few weeks after, and involved all or part of the originally denervated area. According to these workers, the pains were exactly comparable, at least in one case, to thalamic pains and were accompanied by hyperpathia.

Falconer (1953) reported on his experience of treating phantom limb pain by cordotomy. In six cases of upper phantom limb pain he performed cervical cordotomy: in three of these patients there was some recovery of sensibility in the trunk and in the lower limb rendered analgesic by the operation, and continued and repeated pain stimuli applied to these parts gave rise to irritating and burning sensations; in the fourth case the amputation stump became "very sensitive" and objected "strongly to any pressure." In six cases of lower phantom limb pain Falconer performed thoracic cordotomy; one patient complained of a "continuous sensation of pins-and-needles in the phantom foot."

Zülch and Schmid (1953) reported the onset, in a patient subjected to dorsal cordotomy at D5, of a hyperpathia to pricking stimuli, deep pressure, and cutaneous stimuli in the analgesic area.

Roulhac (1953) reported no paresthesias or central pains in a series of 12 cases subjected to bilateral operation.

Falconer (1955) in a personal communication to White and Sweet reported the onset of a burning pain below the costal margin on recovery of the pain sense in one side of the body rendered analgesic by cervical cordotomy.

White and Sweet (1955) reported the onset of dysesthesias in the analgesic or hypoalgesic area in eight out of a series of 210 cases and said that they had seen similar complications in two other cases operated on by other surgeons. The onset of "deep aching" or "shooting pains" was observed by these workers in only two cases in a series of over 300 operations; one patient complained of an icy cold sensation which did not diminish until 19 months after operation. According to White and Sweet the most severe paresthesias were observed in patients subjected to cervical cordotomy.

Horrax and Lang (1957), reporting on a series of 50 cases of cordotomy, said that only two patients complained of "burning" dysesthesia in the analgesic area, and they still had it three years after operation.

French (1958), reporting on a series of 121 cervical cordotomies, did not mention the onset of paresthesias or central pains.

Bohm (1960) reported on a series of 73 patients subjected to cordotomy. Out of 39 cases subjected to unilateral or bilateral operation at cervical level, four complained of burning or continuous tingling paresthesia. In four out of 34 cases of bilateral thoracic cordotomy he observed paresthesia in the lower limbs —a sensation of cold, iciness, or burning. In one of these a further cordotomy performed at a higher level raised the pain threshold but did not suppress the burning paresthesia.

White (1963) said that "the complication that constitutes the most serious problem after cordotomy in the individual with long life expectancy is the development of late unpleasant sensory perception in the initially analgesic area." Unpleasant sensory perception was observed in nine out of 50 patients treated with thoracic cordotomy (18 percent) and in four out of 20 treated with cervical cordotomy (20 percent). These unpleasant sensory disturbances were a feeling of glacial cold in the lower limb or foot, burning paresthesias, or dysesthesias. According to White, this syndrome rarely develops in completely analgesic territories. In the case series reported, these phenomena appeared after months of therapeutic success and, in two thirds of the patients, were first observed on recovery of pain sensibility. In only two cases were these dysesthesias severe enough to constitute a "persisting problem." White (1963) stated that in these cases "the burning pain on even light contact with clothing has been as intense as in the thalamic syndrome of Déjerine-Roussy."

Brihaye and Rétif (1961), reporting on 109 operations, observed only one case of allachesthesia accompanied by an intense burning pain in the analgesic territory. The allachesthesia began three days after operation, while the burning sensations began in the analgesic territory three weeks after and lasted until the patient's death four and a half months later.

Sicard *et al.* (1927) reported on the phenomenon of isothermognosis, the condition in which all stimuli applied to the territory affected by cordotomy are perceived as heat.

A peculiar phenomenon that may arise after cordotomy is that of referred pain, known by various terms including allochiria and allachesthesia. Pain and temperature stimuli applied to analgesic or hypoalgesic regions are referred to and perceived by the patient in a part of the affected or contralateral side of the body in which sensibility is normal (Nathan, 1956; Pecker and Le Beau, 1957; Ray and Wolff, 1945; Miserocchi, 1951; Rand, 1960). According to Pecker and Le Beau (1957) this phenomenon may be observed in the case of stimuli other than pain stimuli. The literature that we have been able to consult records some 30 such cases (Nathan, 1956; Miserocchi, 1951; Pecker and Le

Beau, 1957; Holbrock and Gutiérrez-Mahoney, 1947; Ray and Wolff, 1945; White and Sweet, 1955). We have quoted these data because the physiopathological mechanism underlying these phenomena seem to be comparable in some respects to some of the mechanisms that are thought to be responsible for central pain (Nathan, 1956; Pecker and Le Beau, 1957) and because certain of the semeiologic characteristics of referred pains definitely place them on the same level as central pains (unpleasant character, persistence of the sensation after withdrawal of the stimulus, diffusion of the sensation, poor localization, deep pain, etc.).

Discussion

The incidence of central sensory phenomena after anterolateral cordotomy is difficult to evaluate. The cases series reported in the literature, few of which are extensive, include patients suffering from cancer with short postoperative life expectancy and patients suffering from diseases with a long life expectancy. Central sensory phenomena usually appear within a few weeks or months of operation, although there are cases of early onset; hence the incidence of this complication increases in the series relating to cases with a long postoperative survival. In 1955 White and Sweet reported that in a series of 300-odd cordotomies, the majority performed on patients with malignant tumors, the incidence of subjective central phenomena (dysesthesia and pain) was only about 4 to 5 percent; reporting on a series of 70 patients who had a long postoperative survival, White (1963) stated that he observed subjective central phenomena in 18 percent of the thoracic and in 20 percent of the cervical cordotomies. Lapresle and Guiot (1950) observed these phenomena in as many as five out of eight cases in patients suffering from chronic hip joint arthrosis and Siöqvist (1950) reported subjective central phenomena in 11 out of 71 cases, though he did not specify what diseases the patients were suffering from.

To further complicate the problem of evaluating the incidence and significance of these disturbances, not all workers make clear distinctions between dysesthesias, unpleasant sensations, and outright pain.

Can central pains after anterolateral cordotomy be attributed to the lesion of a specific system of fibers? In anterolateral cordotomy not only the spinothalamic fibers themselves are cut but also other ascending-fiber systems concerned with the transmission of pain (spinospinal, spinoreticular, and spinotectal fibers) and ascending- and descending-fiber systems not so concerned (spinocerebellar, pyramidal, and extrapyramidal). The lesion is not pure. However, it may reasonably be said that the lesion responsible must affect the region of the spinal cord in which the so-called spinothalamic tract lies.

It is difficult to see how other fiber systems could be blamed. Indeed, in none of the other operations on the spinal cord which do not interrupt the so-called spinothalamic tract has central pain been observed. Putnam (1933, 1938, 1940), Schürmann (1953), and Oliver (1949), who performed anterior extrapyramidotomies and lateral pyramidotomies for dyskinetic syndromes, operations which do not generally give rise to derangement of temperature and pain sensibility as long as the incisions are not too large, reported no cases of central pains. Only Oliver (1950) specifically mentioned the onset of central pain in one of his patients subjected to cutting of the whole lateral funiculi, an operation which also involves cutting the anterolateral funiculus and which systematically induces controlateral thermoanalgesia. Nor does section of the posterior funiculi produce central pain, as we shall see in the paragraph dealing with posterior cordotomies (p. 78).

It should be remembered that in anterolateral cordotomies the spinothalamic fibers themselves are interrupted as well as the spinoreticular and spinotectal fibers and the fibers of the so-called propriospinal systems or intrinsic systems of the spinal cord.

The interruption of the spinoreticular and spinotectal long fibers intermixed with the spinothalamic fibers proper does not seem to be necessary for the onset of central pain. Indeed, in mesencephalotomies (p. 56) and in thalamotomies (p. 64), operations in which the incidence of central pain is very high, these fibers are almost completely spared. It is therefore reasonable to suppose that central pains from anterolateral cordotomy are due to section of the spinothalamic fibers proper.

In many of the statistics for anterolateral cordotomy results there is no reference to the onset of unpleasant sensory phenomena or outright pain referred to analgesic or hypoalgesic territories lying under the level of the lesion (Leriche, 1937; Babtchine, 1936; Petit-Dutaillis, 1937).

However, many workers report a high incidence of girdle pains more or less at the level of the cordotomy. These pains are usually attributed to root involvement (White and Sweet, 1955). We feel that this type of pain may be of considerable relevance to the problem of central pain. It is probably not simply a root pain, because of involvement of the sensory root outside the spinal cord.

Noordenbos (1959) did not think that girdle pains following anterolateral cordotomy were of radicular origin and put forward a hypothesis to which we shall refer later.

The observations of Ebin (1949) are exceedingly interesting. He treated cases of parkinsonism by sectioning the spinal cord but in a radically different way from anterolateral cordotomy. In his operations (Fig. 23c) the lateral and anterior pyramidal tracts were cut, and the tracts of the posterior funiculi, the spinothalamic tract, and the gray substance of the cord were to some extent involved. He "frequently" observed that pains occurred in the shoulder on the operation side and that they lasted from a few days to several months. They were what are commonly called "root" pains and yet, as Ebin reported, they appeared even when every precaution was taken to avoid damaging the posterior roots. This suggests that they may be the result of a lesion of the posterior root fibers that is inevitably caused "within" the spinal cord. It seems likely that, at least in Ebin's cases, these pains were actually central pains due to lesion of the "paucisynaptic" pathway at the level of the first neuron in the neuraxis, a problem we shall discuss later (p. 146).

SECTION OF THE TRACT OF LISSAUER (FIG. 10)

To our knowledge only Hyndman (1942) and Rand (1960) have performed sections of the fibers of the tract of Lissauer. Hyndman thought that this operation in conjunction with cordotomy would ensure anesthesia at the same level as the section of the anterolateral funiculus. He reached this conclusion on the assumption that the temperature-pain fibers rise four to five segments in the tract of Lissauer before entering the gray substance and synapsing with the secondary neurons. He thought this mode of behavior of the fibers in the tract of Lissauer was the real reason for the level of anesthesia after anterolateral cordotomy being usually four to five dermatomes below the level of the section. Hyndman's experience confirmed his hypothesis: by combining bilateral anterolateral cordotomy at D1 with section of the Lissauer tract on the right he obtained anesthesia at the level of D7 on the left and at D1 on the right. In this patient in dermatomes D1–D5 on the right, the area which according to Hynd-

FIG. 10. Section of the tract of Lissauer, according to Hyndman. The surgical section may go beyond the zone of Lissauer and impinge on the posterior funiculi.

(a) Lissauer's zone; (b) posterior funiculi.

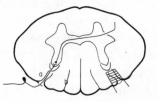

man was rendered analgesic by sectioning Lissauer's tract, there was a reduction of about 25 percent in sensibility to light touch; there were no other disturbances of epicritic sensibility either in these dermatomes or elsewhere. In dermatomes D1–D5 on the right the patient noted a "mild subjective numbness . . . when she rubbed the area with her own hand."

By means of this operation Hyndman obtained areas of anesthesia to temperature and pain extending four to seven dermatomes below the level of the section of the tract of Lissauer in four other cases, which presented no subjective central symptoms.

Rand (1960) combined electrolysis of the tract of Lissauer on the left from C6 to D1 with right cervical cordotomy, which resulted in the phenomenon of referred pain in the right thorax when stimuli were applied to the left thorax.

Discussion

It is impossible to draw conclusions from so small a number of cases, and in any event Hyndman thought it not impossible that section of the tract of Lissauer would involve the adjacent posterior funiculi. Even after this operation subjective central sensory disturbances can still arise in the area depending upon the pain fibers that are probably interrupted: it is thought that a lesion of the first neuron is responsible. (See Fig. 7.)

A very interesting point is that interruption of the tract of Lissauer can result in derangement of the pain sense in bands covering a very large number of dermatomes. In Hyndman's case 4, as may easily be seen by comparing his diagram with Keegan's sensibility diagram (1947) (Fig. 11), hypoesthesia would seem to cover as many as seven dermatomes.

COMMISSURAL MYELOTOMY

The purpose of this operation is to section the temperature-pain fibers originating in the cells of the posterior horns (nucleus proprius and pericornual cells) where they cross on the mid-line at the level of the posterior and anterior commissures in order to obtain bilateral analgesia in the dermatomes corresponding to the fibers cut. The bistoury is introduced posteriorly at the mid-

FIG. 11. One side of a patient subjected to bilateral section of the tract of Lissauer "just above the entrance into the cord of the sixth dorsal posterior root" (on right). The area of anesthesia is bilateral and extends, as shown by the comparison with Keegan's diagram, from dermatomes T5 to T11 inclusive. Within the hatched area sensibility was as follows: pain 0, temperature 50 percent, and light touch 75 percent. This observation would seem to show that the pain fibers may rise as much as six or seven dermatomes in the tract of Lissauer before synapsing with the secondary neurons. *Source:* Hyndman (1942) and Keegan (1947).

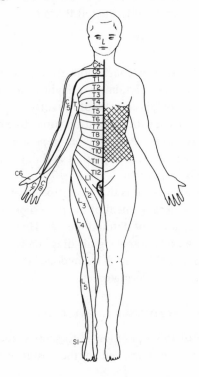

line, splitting the posterior funiculi, and is sunk in order to cut the temperature-pain fibers, which are the only ones that cross the mid-line of the spinal cord (White and Sweet, 1955) (Fig. 12). Armour (1927) first carried out this operation on a patient suffering from tabetic gastric pains; the patient died during the postoperative course.

Putnam (1934) treated three cases of pains in the upper limbs. One of the patients died in the immediate postoperative course. In another the outcome was good: there was anesthesia to temperature and pain stimuli extending from C8 to D10, and there was no loss of deep sensibility in this territory, though there was loss of vibration in the legs; there was no central pain; necropsy disclosed very moderate damage to the dorsal funiculi and a satisfactory division of the commissure. In the third case the result was poor: the pain changed from "sharp," as it had been before operation, to "dull and burning."

Guillaume (1942), reporting on five cases, mentioned no central pain.

Mansuy *et al.* (1944) reported on a series of 30 cases of commissural myelotomy: in only one case did they perform a "total" myelotomy, that is, extending to the anterior commissure; in all the others the incision was 3 mm deep and affected the gray substance. Subjective sensory disturbances, both in the form of

FIG. 12. Diagram of commissural myelotomy. The incision interrupting the spinothalamic fibers while they cross on the mid-line usually covers several metameres. It is made after splitting the posterior funiculi of the cord, which may be contused or injured by incisions that are not dead on the mid-line.

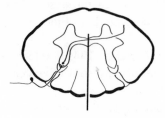

girdle "root" pains in territories corresponding to the myelotomy and in the form of dysesthesia or paresthesia in the lower limbs, were frequently observed. They came on immediately after operation and lasted only 8 to 15 days. The disturbances were observed both in patients who obtained total relief from pain and in those in whom relief was only partial. These workers said that the disturbances may have been due either to traumatic lesions of the roots and cord (which pathways of the cord were not specified!) or to aseptic inflammatory lesions resulting from tiny hemorrhagic effusions due to the operation. Regarding derangement of sensibility, they pointed out that deep sensibility is "practically intact" after this operation; there were objective alterations of sensibility to temperature and pain in only 30 percent of the cases, and these alterations were in the main slight and transient.

Alajouanine and Thurel (1944) reported that they had observed tabetic-type shooting pains after commissural myelotomy.

Guillaume et al. (1945) discussed techniques and indications. They pointed out that during operation the splitting of the posterior funiculi can cause shooting pains but that these disappear with the application of novocaine 10–20 percent. Funicular pains may occur during the postoperative course, but they disappear within a few days. No case series were quoted.

Lhermitte and Puech (1946) performed two commissural myelotomies in a case of phantom limb pains. After the second operation cutaneous hyperalgesia arose in the D5–L3 territory and "pins-and-needles" in the contralateral foot and leg.

David et al. (1947) reported the onset of "so-called sympathetic pains" in the contralateral limb after a commissural myelotomy.

In his monograph Leriche (1949), referring to a commissurotomy, did not mention any subjective central sensory phenomena.

Wertheimer and Sautot (1949) reported on a series of 69 commissurotomies (Mansuy *et al.*, 1944, used part of this material) performed in the majority of cases on patients with pelvic and perineal pain syndromes due to cancer. The data on the site of the incision are not precise: "habituellement centrée . . . sur la 5e vertèbre dorsale" and extending "sur 3 segments médullaires" irrespective of whether the pains radiated to the lower limbs or not. "Parfois (10 cas) l'incision affecta 4 segments médullaires." These workers secured total relief from pain in 29 cases, good results in another 17 cases, and total failure in 13 cases (the authors examined the results of only 59 of the 69 cases treated). They insisted that there was no correlation between the chances of therapeutic success on pain and objective alterations of sensibility to temperature and pain: indeed in only four patients did they obtain temperature-pain anesthesia below the myelotomy and only in 23 patients were appreciable anesthetic areas observed. Deep sensibility was affected in only 11 cases, always slightly and in limited territories. In three cases they observed a "hyperesthésie aux trois modes" (touch-temperature-pain) throughout the territory below the myelotomy. In as many as 18 cases the patients complained during the postoperative course of thoracic girdle pains "systématisées en fonction du siège de l'intervention"; though the pains persisted in two cases, in the majority of cases the pains disappeared after a time. According to the authors, "l'atteinte des cordons postérieurs . . . pourrait en être tenue responsable, l'incision ne respectant pas toujours l'obligation de demeurer strictment médiane."

Wertheimer and Lecuire (1953) reported on a series of 107 cases, in part already discussed by Wertheimer and Sautot (1949). In most of these cases the spinal cord was sectioned at D4, D5, and D6; "root" pains, pains "en ceinture ou évoquant la névralgie intercostale" were observed 27 times and dysesthesia and paresthesia in the lower limbs 28 times. It is interesting that only 21 cases had disturbances of sensibility to light touch (anesthesia, hypesthesia, hyperesthesia); six cases had deep sensibility, and only 30 percent had alterations of temperature and pain sense. There are no data that permit a correlation between site and type of sensibility disturbances on the one hand and girdle pains or dysesthesias of the lower limbs on the other.

Pieri (1951) performed a posterior commissural myelotomy at the level of D3 and D4 in a patient who complained of girdle pains after removal of a subdiaphragmatic neurinoma. The pains disappeared but were replaced by moderate paresthesias in the lower limbs, followed two months later by a sense of agonizing constriction in the lower half of the body with paraparesis. Pieri wondered whether these disturbances might have been due to intraspinal development of the tumor.

Discussion

Central sensory phenomena ranging from outright pain to dysesthesias and paresthesias are fairly frequent after commissural myelotomy but there is considerable doubt as to their interpretation. It is exceedingly difficult to say which systems of fibers are actually interrupted and what the extent of the lesion is in this operation. Wertheimer and Lecuire (1953) emphasized that we know very little about the site and mode of decussation of the spinothalamic fibers. According to some workers decussation occurs at the level at which the posterior root fibers enter the spinal cord; according to others it occurs two segments higher, whereas still others consider that the decussation area is much higher and extends over five or six segments. There is not even agreement as to whether the fibers decussate in the anterior and/or the posterior commissures.

Assuming a wide range of variability in the decussation of the fibers it is clear that a section extending over vertebral bodies D4–D6, corresponding to segments D6–D9 of the spinal cord (Elsberg, 1941), can theoretically interrupt fibers coming from roots D6–L2 and allowing for the fact that the fibers of the posterior roots can rise some segments (as many as four or five, according to Hyndman, 1942) in the tract of Lissauer before ending in the posterior horns, it is obvious that such an incision may interrupt fibers coming from levels even below L2. Yet, to reach the commissure of the cord one must split the posterior funiculi, which are inevitably contused and may be damaged, as anatomic controls have shown; moreover, sometimes the incision is not dead on the mid-line.

True pains have been reported only at the level of the operation, roughly speaking, and are girdle pains. According to Wertheimer and Sautot (1949), they may be due to involvement of the posterior funiculi. It seems rather strange that these pains could be due to this mechanism when one considers that on the mid-line of the thoracic spinal cord the posterior funiculi gather up the fibers coming from the lower limbs but not from thoracic segments. It does, however, seem likely that the lesion of the posterior funiculi is responsible for dysesthesias and paresthesias of the lower limbs. We would emphasize here that these disturbances do not appear to be true pain, at least judging from the data of workers who have had large case series and who distinguish them sharply from the girdle or band pains found at thoracic level (Wertheimer and Lecuire, 1953). Perhaps band pains are due to section of prematurely decussating spinothalamic fibers coming from dermatomes corresponding to the level of section or to genuine root damage. However, one must consider the case of Lhermitte and Puech (1946) in which cutaneous hyperalgesia arose in territory D5–L3. This distribution of hyperalgesia may, on the basis of the above anatomical considerations, correspond to the areas of origin of spinothalamic fibers decussating at various levels in the spinal cord: the hyperalgesia was probably due to lesion of the spinothalamic system.

The only workers who speak of true pains on stimulation of the posterior funiculi are Guillaume et al. (1945), who said that they had observed them as a result of splitting of the funiculi. Actually, it is not clear whether they were pains due to stimulation of the funiculi proper or of the pia that invests them. White and Sweet (1955), quoting the data of Guillaume *et al.* on page 238 of their book, stated: "In our experience the pia over the posterior columns is extremely sensitive to tactile stimuli. If the patient complains of pain, this can be controlled by a brief application of a cotton pledget soaked in 2 percent procaine."

BULBAR SPINOTHALAMIC TRACTOTOMY (FIG. 13)

White (1941) reported a case of spinothalamic tractotomy at bulbar level: there was no central pain.

Schwarz and O'Leary in 1941 and 1942 reported two cases of this operation, one patient dying two days and the other 29 days after the operation. These workers did not report central pain.

Crawford (1947) treated 11 patients. He reported no central pain.

Klemme (1949) treated nine patients suffering from pain syn-

FIG. 13. Diagram of spinothalamic tractotomy at bulbar level. Cross-section of the superior part of the bulb. The surgical incision (framed area) interrupting the spinothalamic tract may impinge upon adjacent reticular structures and the descending tract of V. In the spinothalamic tract at this level, not only are the spinothalamic fibers proper interrupted but also the spinotectal and spinoreticular fibers united to them. The medial lemniscus tract at this level is usually completely spared. *Source:* White and Sweet (1955).

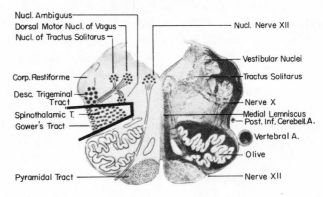

50

dromes of tumoral and non-tumoral origin, one with a bilateral operation. He made a 3-mm-deep section (other workers have gone as deep as 6 mm). He reported no paresthesias or central pain.

D'Errico (1950) performed 12 bulbar spinothalamic tractotomies for pains in the neck, shoulders, and upper limbs. Neither paresthesia nor central pain was observed in any of the patients.

Crawford and Knighton (1953) reported eight cases, in one of which central dysesthesia (burning sensation) arose all over the body. In three cases the lesion extended backward, involving the descending root of the trigeminal nerve.

Zülch and Schmid (1953) reported the case of a patient subjected to cordotomy of the spinothalamic tract at the level of the upper limit of emergence of the radicles of XI, with resulting analgesia from D3 downward in the contralateral half of the body and simultaneously a high degree of hyperpathia to deep pressure; furthermore, the incision went too far backward, thereby causing mild homolateral trigeminal hypesthesia.

They also reported a second case, in which a Siöqvist trigeminal tractotomy was performed, with resulting homolateral trigeminal hypesthesia and a high degree of hyperpathia; on the contralateral side there was analgesia and hyperpathia for deep pressure from C4 together with burning pains precipitated by light touch and vibration stimuli. The authors considered that these disturbances were a result of the fact that the surgical lesion had gone too far forward and partially interrupted the spinothalamic tract.

Adams and Munro (1944) treated three cases of pain due to tumor, performing a bilateral operation in one case. Necropsy was done in all three cases. In two cases the wound extended to within 2 to 3 mm of the mid-line, while in the third case it was 5 to 6 mm deep; the spinothalamic tract was cut but the medial lemniscus was spared, apart from a few ventral fibers in one case. Judging from the spinal cord sections reproduced and from the authors' explicit statement, one can only conclude that the "lateral reticular substance" also was affected by the lesion. Sensibility tests revealed thermoanalgesia on the contralateral side from D2 (the most medial fibers of the spinothalamic tract seem to have been spared) and in one case a mild tactile hypesthesia. There were no dysesthesias or central pains or derangement of epicritic sensibility in any of the cases. According to these workers it is impossible to section the cervical portion of the spinothalamic tract at bulbar level without injuring other systems.

White and Sweet (1955) reported two cases of bulbar tractotomy in which contralateral analgesia was replaced five years later by "a capacity to distinguish pin-point from pin-head." In one case a "slight spreading 'irritating sensation' in the region of the prick was experienced" and "a test tube filled with ice now caused this same type of sensation without a feeling of cold in the previously analgesic thermanaesthetic area." In the other patient "a pinprick felt like a spreading, deep, uncomfortable feeling in the general area near the point when applied almost anywhere in the previously analgesic zone." In neither of the two cases was there "a disagreeable quality in the stimulus of touch in these regions." These workers also reported that they had observed a case of paresthesia in the homolateral half of the face because the section had impinged on the descending tract of the trigeminal.

Sweet et al. (1960) reported the results of a method of coagulation of the spinothalamic tract. After occipital craniectomy the coagulating electrode is fixed at the level of the obex immediately in front of the point of emergence of the radicles of XI. This method was used on eight cases of pain from cancer. In two cases pains appeared during the postoperative course in previously unaffected areas on the homolateral side. In one of these cases the cut had overstepped the mid-line, as shown by a histologic section of the bulb. The authors did not comment on this. Necropsy was not done in the other case, and there are no data for the tumor site. It must not be forgotten, however, that these two patients had metastases and pain may possibly have been due to these. There is no mention of epicritic sensibility deficit; from the case records it would seem that these pathways were untouched. Sections of the bulb are reproduced in six cases but there is no comment on the formations of the cord destroyed by the lesion apart from the spinothalamic tract. In any case, there is no reference to central pain.

Zülch (1960) quoted no cases but stated that after bulbar spinothalamic tractotomy central pain (hyperpathia) may arise, reiterating his conviction that this is due to incomplete lesions of the spinothalamic tract which only reduce the number of its fibers.

Crawford (1960) treated four patients: one was suffering from phantom limb pain; a measure of anesthesia at C1 was obtained at first but this was followed by a "painful anesthesia" syndrome; in another patient "psychogenic" pains appeared in sites other than that of the original pain.

Birkenfeld and Fisher (1963) treated a case of causalgia successfully; no central pains appeared.

Discussion

It is rare for central pain and related phenomena to occur after bulbar spinothalamic tractotomy: only Zülch and Schmid (1953) and Crawford (1960) reported definite cases. This operation has been performed only a few times (about 60), mostly in cancer cases with short life expectancy. This may well be one of the reasons for the low incidence of central pain and related phenomena after this operation.

At the bulbar level the spinothalamic fibers are interrupted as well as the spinotectal fibers (which at bulbar level still run together with the spinothalamic fibers [Peele, 1954]) and the spinoreticular fibers which are still united to the spinothalamic tract and have not yet ended in the reticular formations of the brainstem. The spinothalamic/spinoreticular/spinotectal contingent is fairly superficial at this level and therefore easy to attack. Interruption can thus be total or subtotal and the lesion is fairly "pure." However, as Adams and Munro (1944) stated, it is difficult to interrupt even the contingent of fibers originating at cervical levels without damaging other fiber systems. Furthermore, if the incision goes too deep the reticular formations of the bulb are liable to injury. Only a few cases have been controlled histologically, but Crawford and Knighton (1953) observed in one of their patients not only complete destruction of the spinothalamic tract but also damage to the surrounding reticular areas. In the material of White and Sweet (1955) and of Sweet *et al.* (1960), there were cases in which the lesions definitely involved the reticular structures of the bulb. But it does not seem that central sensory phenomena occurred in any of these cases.

Actually, it is not unusual for the lesion to extend to the reticular structures of the bulb. On the other hand, the tracts and nuclei of Goll and Burdach, which are separated from the spinothalamic tract by the descending root of the trigeminal, are fairly consistently spared. Furthermore, the higher the section, the less likely it is that the medial lemniscus will be affected, because the bulbothalamic neurons cross and go on to the mid-line far from the surgical incision.

Section of the spinothalamic tract at bulbar level, which is performed 0–6 mm below the obex, interrupts not only the spinothalamic fibers proper (the paucisynaptic system or neospinothalamic according to Mehler, 1957), but also the spinoreticular fibers, which belong to the so-called polysynaptic (or paleospinothalamic) system. It is important to remember, as do Albe-Fessard and Fessard (1963), that "a large part of the fibers with reticular termination stop at the bulbar level. There they synapse with the cells of the nucleus reticularis gigantocellularis." In all likelihood, the surgical lesion made at bulbar level is usually below this nucleus gigantocellularis of the reticular formation and probably interrupts the majority of the ascending fibers ending in the reticular formation. This is clearly seen in Fig. 14, which shows the site of the nucleus gigantocellularis of Olszewski (1954) and the site of the incision made in bulbar spinothalamic tractotomy according to White and Sweet (1955). Moreover, the nucleus gigantocellularis and "the bulbar reticular formation constitute the principal relay of the extra-lemniscal pathway leading to the center median-parafascicular complex" and the center median nucleus is activated by "stimuli which deserve the designation of noxious" (Albe-Fessard and Fessard, 1963).

It is not unlikely that the low incidence of central pain secondary to this operation is due to the fact that it interrupts not only the paucisynaptic contingent of the spinothalamic tract but also to a large extent the spinoreticulothalamic polysynaptic system, since the surgical incision interrupts the spinoreticular fibers which run intermingled with the spinothalamic fibers before they separate off to reach the nucleus gigantocellularis. It

FIG. 14. Diagram of the brainstem in superolateral view. The spinothalamic tractotomy incision shown at (e) interrupts the true spinothalamic fibers and a very large percentage of the spinoreticular fibers united with them. A large number of these fibers end in the nucleus gigantocellularis of Olszewski, which forms part of the reticular formation of the bulb and which according to Albe-Fessard and Fessard (1963) constitutes the main relay of an extralemniscal sensory pathway "leading to the center median parafascicular complex" concerned with the transmission of nociceptive impulses.

(a) Pons; (b) IV ventricle; (c) olivary body; (d) nucleus gigantocellularis of Olszewski; (e) the spinothalamic tractotomy incision made at bulbar level.

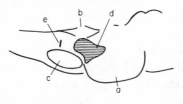

may also be related to the fact that, as we have seen from the anatomical data, the incision usually extends well into the reticular formation.

OPERATIONS AT PONS LEVEL

Serra and Neri (1936) treated a case of facial pains from tumor of the base of the skull by electrocoagulation of the sensory nucleus of the trigeminal performed at the level of the pons at the point where the trigeminal radicles enter the neuraxis. They did not report the onset of central pain.

Clovis Vincent carried out coagulation of the quintothalamic tract in the rostral portion of the pons in eight cases; four patients survived. In no cases were central sensory phenomena observed.

Discussion

The material is too limited to permit any conclusions.

SPINOTHALAMIC TRACTOTOMY AT MESENCEPHALIC LEVEL;
MEDIAL MESENCEPHALOTOMY

Open Lateral Mesencephalotomy (*Spinothalamic Tractotomy*) (Fig. 15). Dogliotti (1938) effected electrocoagulation of the spinothalamic tract in the upper portion of the pons and the lowest part of the midbrain in four patients. One patient died within 36 hours; in two other patients complete contralateral analgesia was obtained but "unpleasant dysesthesias" appeared soon afterward. Unfortunately, we have not seen the details of this report and so cannot say whether the epicritic sensibilities were affected.

Walker (1942a) treated two cases—one of testicular teratoma with cervical and abdominal metastases and one of phantom limb pain in the arm—with mesencephalic tractotomy. In the first case paresthesias and hyperpathia appeared on the treated side during the third week. In the other case burning paresthesias came on a few days after operation; there was deficit of sensibility to light touch, which was demonstrated only by testing with Frey's hairs.

Guiot and Forjaz (1947) performed two lateral mesencephalotomies. Tactile and deep sensibility were intact in both cases; in one there was complete contralateral hemianesthesia to temperature and pain, whereas in the other the analgesic area was circumscribed (these workers stated that they performed a selective mesencephalotomy). No central sensory phenomena occurred in either of these patients.

FIG. 15. Diagram of open lateral mesencephalic tractotomy and corresponding histologic section. The surgical section that here interrupts almost electively the spinothalamic fibers proper (since the spinoreticular and some of the spinotectal fibers have already been arrested at lower levels) may impinge on the reticular formation of the midbrain and the medial lemniscus.

(A) Aquaeductus Sylvii; (S) tractus spinothalamicus; (M) lemniscus medialis; (I) brachium colliculi inferioris. *Source:* Walker (1942a).

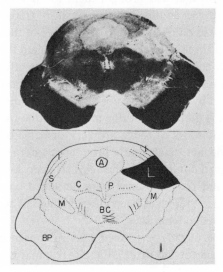

David *et al.* (1947) performed a lateral mesencephalotomy in a 75-year-old patient suffering from postherpetic neuralgia in the territory of the brachial plexus. The patient, who died three days later, did not suffer either from paresthesias or from central pains. It appears that epicritic sensibility was normal.

Siöqvist (1949) reported on two lateral mesencephalotomy cases, one of whom died on the seventh and the other on the tenth day; neither patient seems to have suffered from central pains.

Walker (1950), reviewing his own material, reported that of 12 patients surviving 10 percent had paresthesias.

Schwarz (1950) observed disagreeable paresthesias in two cases of lateral mesencephalotomy.

Drake and MacKenzie (1953) performed six mesencephalotomies. Within 3 to 14 days of operation all the patients experienced subjective sensory phenomena: "unbearable" and "entirely new" sensations brought on by pricking, deep pressure, and heat stimuli. In three cases spontaneous burning pains appeared; in two patients the pains extended throughout half the body on the treated side though they were more intense in the site of the pain that had brought them to operation; and in the third the pain was confined to this territory (face). The authors stated that these pains were similar to those of the thalamic syndrome. In all three patients there was complete thermoanalgesia on the side that had been treated and that was affected by dysesthesias, and all complained of a very mild hypesthesia to light touch, elicited by the cotton wool test. The mildness of the tactile disturbances is thought to be due to the fact that the central fibers subserving the sense of touch are very dispersed, hence a small incision could not determine a pronounced derangement of this sense. Standard clinical tests showed that deep sensibility, vibration sense, and position sense were deranged only in one case, but in this case there had been clear damage of the cerebral peduncle and medial lemniscus.

Bailey *et al.* (1954) performed a lateral mesencephalotomy in a case of cancer of the external auditory canal extending to the face and cervical plexus. They obtained hypoalgesia throughout the side contralateral to the section with the exception of the mandibular branch of V, which became hyperalgesic to pricking and to light contact with cotton wool; there were no definite signs of deficit of epicritic sensibility except for a doubtful proprioceptive loss in the upper limb. In commenting on their case Bailey *et al.* stated that the trigeminal hyperalgesia was "surely" due to infiltration of the trigeminal fibers by the tumor. They also carried out a detailed anatomical study of the case: the surgical section had caused degeneration not only of the spinothalamic tract but also of the medial lemniscus, lateral lemniscus, and brachium conjunctivum, supraoptic and posterior commissures, and spinohypothalamic fibers. An interesting point is that at this level the fibers of the spinothalamic tract are mixed "perhaps with the fibers of the medial lemniscus," but nevertheless the authors emphasized the fact that in their case the deficit attributable to lesion of the medial lemniscus was clinically very slight.

Mikula *et al.* (1959) performed a bilateral lateral mesencephalotomy in a single operation on a tabetic who suffered from attacks of gastric pain. They obtained analgesia to temperature and pain throughout the body without loss of tactile or deep sensibility and the attacks of pain ceased. About seven days after operation, however, the patient began to complain of "pins-and-needles" all over the body, which gave him a "disagreeable impression that hurts."

Morello (1962) did not report any central pains after lateral mesencephalotomy.

Stereotactic Mesencephalotomy (*Spinothalamic Tractotomy and Medial Mesencephalotomy*) (Fig. 16). Torvik (1959) reported on two stereotactic spinothalamic tractotomies. In the first patient, who was suffering from lung cancer, histologic examination showed that the lesion had completely destroyed the spinothalamic tract and medial lemniscus, had partially destroyed the reticular formation of the brainstem and brachium of the inferior colliculus, but had only begun to encroach on the red nucleus and superior colliculus. The patient had presented thermoanalgesia in the arms and legs, thermohypoalgesia in the trunk and forehead, and very mild thermohypoalgesia around the mouth; there was also a fair degree of tactile deficit, though this was retained to some extent even in the limbs. Hyperpathia to pain (pinching) and vibration stimuli arose during the postoperative course. In the second case the lesion involved the spi-

FIG. 16. Section of the brainstem made through the anterior portion of the posterior commissure. According to Spiegel and Wycis the lesion of the spinothalamic tract during stereotactic mesencephalotomy is usually made at this level. At this level the true spinothalamic fibers are interrupted almost exclusively, since the spinotectal and spinoreticular fibers have mostly already left the spinothalamic tract. However, the stereotactic lesion usually impinges on the reticular formation of the midbrain and on the medial lemniscus.

(R) Red nucleus; (Ni) substantia nigra; (FH) Forel's field; (Gm) medial geniculate body; (pr) pretectal region; (pu) pulvinar; (Spt + ml) spinothalamic tract and medial lemniscus. *Source:* Spiegel and Wycis (1953).

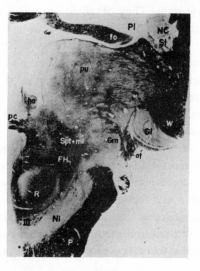

nothalamic tract and medial lemniscus and extended to the most medial portion of the thalamus. This patient survived only 14 days, but no central pains appeared during that time.

Mazars *et al.* (1959, 1960) reported on 86 stereotactic operations for coagulation of the spinothalamic tract at mesencephalic level. In no case did they observe central pain.

Wycis and Spiegel (1962) observed dysesthesias in eight out of 54 lateral mesencephalotomies (14.8 percent). They were very severe in two cases only; however, the disturbances were transient in one case only. The surgical lesion involved not only the spino- and quintothalamic tracts but also a large part of the adjacent reticular substance at the level of the posterior colliculi. They gave no precise data on loss of epicritic sensibility. The same workers (1953) stated in a paper on six cases that sensory disturbances might arise after stereotactic mesencephalotomy through lesion of the medial lemniscus but that they were mild and always transient (Spiegel and Wycis, 1953).

Roeder and Orthner (1961) reported data that deserve particular attention. They treated a case of trigeminal painful anesthesia resulting from alcoholic injection of the gasserian ganglion, by stereotactic mesencephalotomy. Their intention had been to attack the reticular formation and not the long spino- and quintothalamic pathways; according to these workers, the coagulation interrupted the reticular substance of the anterior portion of the midbrain, while the spinothalamic tract and medial lemniscus were essentially ("im Wesentlichen") spared. The facial pain disappeared and the cheek was anesthetic; hypesthesia to light touch and pain arose on one side of the body and hypesthesia to heat in the leg; vibration and position sense were practically unaffected. At follow-up eight months after operation there was still facial anesthesia and hypoalgesia on the right side of the body, although stimulation with cotton wool and tuning fork and often even lying on the right side aroused unpleasant paresthesias. This hyperpathia—or so the authors called it— affected the right side of the face, the maxilla, the right arm, and the inner half of the leg. The patient was pleased with the result and said that the disturbances were bearable. The authors did not carry out an anatomical examination of the surgical lesion. As we have seen, they said that the spinothalamic tract was "essentially" spared. In our view, however, the onset of hypoalgesia on the contralateral half of the body clearly shows that this pathway was affected.

Discussion

Of all operations designed to suppress pain open spinothalamic tractotomy at mesencephalic level seems to have the highest incidence of subjective central sensory phenomena (dysesthesias and pains). These phenomena are likely to occur in a substantial percentage of cases even in stereotactic mesencephalotomy: in the case series of Wycis and Spiegel (1962), which is one of the largest, they occurred in 14.8 percent of the cases, and yet in the 86 cases of Mazars *et al.* (1959, 1960) there is no reference to them.

At mesencephalic level the spinothalamic tract lies near the surface and is easy to attack; it should therefore be easy to make a relatively "pure" section of this system. In fact, however, at this level the spinotectal fibers are injured together with the spinothalamic fibers and even the medial lemniscus fibers are apt to be involved, for, according to Rasmussen and Peyton (1948), the fibers of the medial lemniscus lie partly dorsal to the lateral sulcus of the midbrain, and according to Bailey *et al.* (1954) perhaps a few of the medial lemniscus fibers are intermingled with those of the spinothalamic tract.

Actually, few workers refer to epicritic loss after open operations for lateral mesencephalotomy and usually the disturbances are mild, inconstant, and transient (Walker, 1942a; Drake and MacKenzie, 1953; Bailey *et al.,* 1954). There is probably greater risk of involving the medial lemniscus in stereotactic operations because the lesions are larger. These deficits are rarely alluded to in these operations, and only Torvik (1959) gave a clear description of extensive lesions on the medial lemniscus.

According to Noordenbos (1959) "damage to the medial lemniscus . . . is almost certain" even in open lateral mesencephalotomy.

From this point of view mesencephalic spinothalamic tractotomy differs from tractotomies performed at lower levels of the neuraxis, which are less likely to result in damage to the epicritic sensibility system. At spinal cord level the tracts of Goll and Burdach are far from the site of the incision, whereas at bulbar level the epicritic pathways are separated from the spinothalamic tract by the descending root of the trigeminal and in the upper portions of the bulb they already begin to decussate on the mid-line. It is difficult to say whether this risk of simultaneous damage to the epicritic pathways, even if not constant and not always documented, is of importance in the causation of central pains. It is worth remembering that after stereotactic mesencephalotomies, which are more likely to injure the pathway of epicritic sensibility as well as the reticular formation of the midbrain, as we shall shortly see, the onset of central pain seems to be less frequent than after open operations.

Midbrain lesions invariably extend to the adjacent reticular formations both in open operations (Fig. 15) and in stereotactic operations (see Torvik, 1959) (Fig. 16). Some workers go so far as to extend the lesion to the reticular formation deliberately (Roeder and Orthner, 1961), while others take it for granted that this formation will be involved (Wycis and Spiegel, 1962). This extension of the lesion may well be relevant to the pathogenesis of central pain.

Another important feature of mesencephalic spinothalamic tractotomies which we believe might be highly relevant to the problem of the physiopathology of central pain is this: at midbrain level the spinothalamic tract consists of only a small number of fibers, about 1500 according to Glees and Bailey (1951), and a very high percentage of the fibers of the anterolateral funiculus of the spinal cord, which similarly subserve the transmission of pain, have stopped at the level of the reticular formations of the lower portion of the brainstem (spinoreticular fibers); moreover, the collaterals of the fibers severed at mesencephalic level may still convey pain impulses on the polysynaptic systems of the spinal cord and brainstem. In other words, after this operation a very large quantity of pain impulses may still converge on the subthalamic polysynaptic systems and via these systems be transmitted to higher levels (Fig. 6).

STEREOTACTIC THALAMOTOMIES (FIG. 17)

Hassler and Riechert (1959) stated that the onset of central pain after stereotactic operations with destruction of the sensory nuclei of the thalamus was a rare phenomenon. They observed central sensory phenomena in only one of 24 cases treated stereotactically. This patient had been suffering from phantom limb pain; the ventral sensory nuclei (VPL and VPM) were coagulated, with resulting anesthesia on the contralateral side of

FIG. 17. Schematic drawing of the thalamus. Stereotactic lesions aimed at the VPM and VPL nuclei are likely to overstep the target and impinge on the formations belonging to the diffuse projection system: the CM nucleus and the Lamina Medullaris Interna.

VPM, VPL: nuclei Ventro Postero Medial and Ventro Postero Lateral; LMI: Lamina Medullaris Interna; CM: Center Median Nucleus; GB: Globus Pallidus.

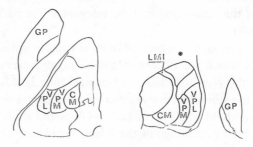

the body, less marked in the trigeminal area. Six weeks after operation, when the sensory deficit caused by it was regressing, a thalamic syndrome appeared.

Mark *et al.* (1960) performed 17 stereotactic thalamotomies. Central sensory phenomena, mostly confined to a feeling of numbness, occurred in three patients. When discussing their results, these workers stated that in only one case did the painful dysesthesias constitute a real problem and that a new lesion through an indwelling electrode stopped the pain. They consider that their method affords some guarantee of avoiding thalamic pain because the coagulating electrodes are left *in situ;* hence, further coagulations can be effected by extending the lesions in order to block the pain. We have been unable to identify in the case list the patient in question; in any case, in this patient the electrode had been left in the VPL.

Mark *et al.* (1963) in a later paper studied the extent of stereotactic lesions. They observed that in the majority of cases the lesions impinged not only on the specific relay nuclei (VPL and VPM) but also on the nuclei of the diffuse projection system (center median and parafascicular).

Bettag and Yoshida (1960), who treated seven cases of painful facial anesthesia by thalamic coagulation operations, said that in four cases (three treated with lesion of the arcuate nucleus and one with lesion of the center median and dorsomedial nuclei), after an 8 to 12 week period without pain, pains returned, but they were different from the previous pains and were of the nature of dysesthesia. No specific mention is made of thalamic pain, however; in all cases the pains were confined to the trigeminal area of the face and were described as a feeling of burning, pricking, stiffness, "pins-and-needles," and tingling. The authors reported no data on sensory deficits due to operation on the side of the body contralateral to the lesion.

Riechert (1961) stated that the onset of central pain after stereotactic thalamotomy is a dreaded but relatively rare occurrence. Wycis (1961) disputed this statement and said that he preferred to perform mesencephalotomy stereotactically because there is less risk of central pain.

Obrador *et al.* (1961) treated a case of phantom limb pain by destroying the VPL and dorsomedial nuclei. The phantom limb pain disappeared and hypesthesia to touch-temperature-pain stimuli appeared on one side of the body. Pain stimuli "tienen un cierto caracter disestesico."

In our experience (Cassinari *et al.*, 1963a and b, 1964, Maspes and Pagni, 1965, Pagni, 1966) out of 32 cases of stereotactic thalamotomy for pain syndromes central pain was observed in six cases (18 percent). The target area for coagulation was as follows: in three cases (nos. 1, 2, 3) the VPL, VPM, and center median nuclei; in one case (no. 4) the VPL nucleus, Reil's band (medial lemniscus) at subthalamic level, and the center median nucleus; in one case (no. 5) the center median nucleus only (see Appendix p. 159).

The immediate result in regard to the pains for which the patients came to operation was very good in all five cases. Furthermore, in all five cases there was more or less severe sensory loss to all modalities on the side contralateral to the surgical lesion.

In case 1 central pain appeared one and a half months after operation and lasted until his death five months later. The pains affected a larger area than had those for which the patient was operated on but they included this area.

In case 2 central pain appeared on the 13th day after operation and lasted until death occurred on the 56th day; the pain affected the entire half of the body, including the face and extended beyond the area covered by the pains which brought the patient to operation.

In case 3 central pain appeared on the sixth day and disappeared on the 21st day; the patient had no relapse of the pains for which he was operated on; hyperpathia extended throughout one half of the body, including the face.

In case 4 central pain appeared on the eighth day and still persists at 16 months after operation; it is more extensive than the original pains. In this case it is difficult to say whether the pain that returned in the site of the original pain was solely central pain or a true relapse of the original pain.

In case 5 central pain appeared on the eighth day and still persists after four months; it covers a large area and affects also the face, the site of the pains for which the patient was operated on.

There is one very interesting point in connection with case 3, operated on for postrhizotomy trigeminal painful anesthesia: central pain affected the whole of one side of the body or covered a very large area except the affected side of the face, which had been denervated by the rhizotomy. In the other three cases (nos. 1, 2, 4) in which the area of the pains for which the patients had been operated on was not denervated or only partially so the pain affected these districts also.

The last case (no. 6) in this series is considered separately. In this patient, in whom the target area was the center median nucleus, the first coagulation resulted in cessation of the facial pains (due to a growth) without sensory loss. Because of partial relapse of the pain a second coagulation was effected, this time centering on the VPM: the spontaneous pains disappeared but sensory disturbances appeared on the affected side of the body and with them central pain not affecting the face. In this patient there had been trigeminal hypesthesia in the pain territory before the two operations.

Along with this series of thalamic pains due to a stereotactic lesion effected for the treatment of pain syndromes, we would record another personal observation (no. 7) of a patient suffering from facial paraspasm. The right center median nucleus was coagulated, as Bettag and Rottgen (1961) had done. There was only temporary relief of the paraspasm and on the tenth day the patient began to complain of spontaneous dysesthesias on the left side of the face and in the left hand. Stimulation of these two regions precipitated a certain amount of pain. Clinical testing showed hypesthesia to all modalities in the third and fourth fingers of the left hand and all stimuli applied to the left side of the face were felt "pervertedly." These phenomena are unchanged at seven months from operation.

Discussion

Many workers have performed stereotactic operations on the sensory nuclei of the thalamus for pain syndromes (Hecaen *et al.,* 1949; Monnier and Fisher, 1951; Talairach *et al.,* 1955; Laspiur, 1956; Hassler, 1958; Hassler and Riechert, 1959; Bettag and Yoshida, 1960; Mark *et al.,* 1960; Jouvet *et al.,* 1960; Hankinson *et al.,* 1960; Obrador and Bravo, 1960; Bettag, 1961; Riechert, 1961; Obrador *et al.,* 1961; Cassinari *et al.,* 1963, Maspes and Pagni, 1965; Pagni, 1966). The majority of these operations were performed to relieve thalamic pain due to vascular insult. In the other cases, according to Riechert (1961), the onset of thalamic pain due to the surgical lesion is a rare occurrence. But, as we have seen from our experience (Cassinari *et al.,* 1963a and b, Maspes and Pagni, 1965, Pagni, 1966), this is not an infrequent occurrence. Lesions centering on the relay nuclei of the thalamus (VPL and VPM) sever the medial lemniscus and the spinothalamic fibers and spare the contingent of spinoreticular fibers and the polysynaptic systems that are distributed all over the brainstem. Thus, as in mesencephalotomy, an enormous quantity of pain impulses is still transmitted via the polysynaptic systems to the brainstem-thalamic structures that some workers consider to be of such great importance in the conscious perception of pain.

This, however, is not the complete story. There is no doubt that with the techniques currently employed the lesions also cut a very high percentage of the fibers of epicritic sensibility at thalamic level (as proved by the severe epicritic deficits resulting from these operations) and the thalamoparietal tertiary neurons. As far as we know, there are no cases in the literature of anatomically controlled stereotactic lesions in which only the pain fibers were damaged, that is to say cases in which a very circumscribed elective lesion destroyed only the parvicellular ventrocaudal nucleus of Hassler, that is, the thalamic relay nucleus of the pain fibers. Even Hassler and Riechert (1959), who say that they identify this nucleus by electrical stimulation, reported cases in which the lesion went well beyond its limits. It would be exceedingly interesting to have cases of this type because then the question as to whether a concomitant lesion of the epicritic pathways is necessary for the onset of central pain would be answered once and for all. Moreover, this would actually be impossible if, as some workers think, the pain and epicritic fibers are superimposed at thalamic level.

Not even the case of Hoffmann (1933), in which the extremely circumscribed lesion was confined to the most basal part of the posterior ventral nucleus of the thalamus, that is, the parvicellular ventrocaudal nucleus, and in which there was a typical thalamic syndrome due to a vascular lesion, the case that Hassler (1960) regarded as the one with the smallest anatomically controlled thalamic lesion to date, does not yield the final answer. Indeed, although "touch," vibration, shapes (circles, crosses, lines), and the texture of different materials were correctly perceived on the affected side, the presence of a "classic astereognosis" of the hand suggests that the thalamic lesion went beyond the specific pain relay nucleus.

There is another important point in connection with stereotactic lesions of the thalamus: however hard one may try to confine the lesions to the sensory nuclei they always impinge on the nuclei of the diffuse projection system of the thalamus immediately adjacent to the sensory relay nuclei. This is clearly established by the histopathologic data of Mark *et al.* (1962, 1963) and of Maspes and Pagni (1965). Even on the basis of the macroscopical data that can be deduced from the figures published by Hassler and Riechert (1959), it is clear that, although the lesions were centered on the posterior ventral nuclei, they went beyond these toward the reticular formation of the thalamus (external reticular nucleus) and toward the intralaminar nuclei. This encroachment of the lesions on the diffuse projection systems is probably of importance in the genesis of central pain, either as a promoting factor or perhaps as a factor limiting its onset.

Material we feel is important because it enables us to state that a lesion of the sensory nuclei is absolutely necessary for the onset of thalamic pain is as follows. In the collective experience of workers throughout the world, which now numbers thousands of cases, stereotactic lesions made in the thalamic nuclei outside the sensory relay nuclei, that is, in the ventrolateral, dorso-medial, anterior, and posterior lateral nuclei (lesions which nec-essarily encroach on the diffuse projection nuclei) have never caused central pain. It may be that a stereotactic lesion aimed at the VL or CM thalamic nuclei impinges on a smaller portion of the VPL nucleus; but it is known that a very small lesion of the VPL and VPM nuclei does not necessarily produce any sensory deficit (Macchi *et al.*, 1964, Pagni *et al.*, 1965). Only if the spe-cific sensory nuclei lesion (VPL–VPM) is large enough to give objective sensory deficit of the contralateral side of the body can central pain and subjective sensory phenomena follow the tha-lamic lesion. In our experience, for instance, lesions centering on the center median nucleus have not caused central pain unless they encroached (see cases 6 and 7 of our case series and Maspes and Pagni, 1965) on the sensory nuclei. The experience of Guiot (1964) is also very interesting in this regard: he also coagulates the thalamic posterior lateral nucleus (LP) in parkinsonism and has never observed central pain.

SUBCORTICAL OPERATIONS: STEREOTACTIC DESTRUCTION OF
THE THALAMOPARIETAL RADIATIONS

Talairach *et al.* (1960) and Riechert *et al.* (1961) (Fig. 18) did not report central pain after destruction of the thalamoparietal radiations in their case series.

Cassinari *et al.* (1963b, 1964) destroyed the thalamoparietal radiations with radioactive yttrium in two cases. In one patient (see Appendix, case 8), suffering from causalgia from tearing of the brachial plexus with total sensory and motor paralysis of the upper limb, the pain being confined to the ulnar aspect of the hand and forearm, central pain appeared. After a three-month period of complete freedom from pain the patient began to have spontaneous new pains all over the upper limb, shoulder, and half of the chest on the same side. These pains were "atrocious," worse than those that brought the patient to operation, and they still persist at 16 months after operation.

PARIETAL CORTECTOMY

We have not found in the literature any cases of central pain arising after parietal cortectomy. Gutiérrez-Mahoney (1944), Horrax (1946), Lhermitte and Puech (1946), David *et al.* (1947), Echols and Colclough (1947), Guitérrez-Mahoney (1948), Wertheimer and Mansuy (1949), Sugar and Bucy (1951), White and Sweet (1955), and Carbonin (1961) have all performed parietal cortectomy for phantom limb pain and postherpetic neuralgia and none of them has reported paresthesias or central pain after the operation. Only Lewin and Phillips (1952) described a case that might be described as postoperative central pain. They performed cortectomy of the posterior lip of the fissure of Rolando in a case of amputation stump pain refractory to local treatment, spinal anesthesia, and cordotomy. The cortectomy re-

FIG. 18. Site and extent of stereotactic lesion made with radioactive yttrium in the thalamoparietal projections during subcortical parietal pain surgery according to Talairach *et al.* (1960). *Source:* adapted from Talairach *et. al.* (1960).

sulted in disappearance of that pain, but five days later there appeared a new pain, quite different from the previous one, and also a feeling of numbness in the ring finger.

It would be interesting to know whether there were any sensory deficits after cortectomy and, if so, of what sort. Unfortunately, the majority of workers concerned did not discuss this point (Gutiérrez-Mahoney, 1944, 1948; Horrax, 1946, case 1; Wertheimer and Mansuy, 1949; Carbonin, 1961).

Not even Talairach *et al.* (1960) in their review of cases of parietal cortectomy for pain syndromes went thoroughly into the problem of sensory losses after this operation. They simply stated that derangement of the pain sense is transient, because the spinothalamic tract has a bilateral connection to the ventro-postero-lateral nuclei with the possibility of replacement by the other hemisphere. These workers also point out that according to Biemond (1956) integration of pain stimuli occurs in the second sensory area.

According to White and Sweet (1955) the sensory deficit that occurs after parietal cortectomy does not include "full-fledged" analgesia.

It is difficult to determine the exact nature of these disturbances partly because cortical resections are generally small and partly because this operation is usually performed in patients with phantom limb pain who have already been subjected to other antalgic operations. In short, the only fairly sure datum that emerges from the literature on parietal cortectomy is that the sensory deficits due to it are more severe at epicritic than at temperature-pain level, though the latter may also be affected.

Discussion

It is rather odd that there is not a single case of definite central pain after parietal cortectomy in the literature and only one case that might perhaps be interpreted as such. It must, however, be borne in mind that most of these operations were performed in cases of phantom limb pain and that the results in such cases are very unsatisfactory. Persisting primary pains may perhaps mask the onset of new pains. Furthermore, if it is true that central pains are generally projected to areas whose pain pathways have been interrupted, it is easy to explain why central pains have never been observed after cortectomy in areas other than the sites of the primary pains, for in these operations every effort has always been made to identify and remove only the area of the cortex corresponding to the sensory projections of the affected limb.

The above considerations are valid if the pain fibers do project to the postcentral gyrus mingled with fibers of epicritic sensibility and if interruption of the paucisynaptic system of pain transmission is necessary for the onset of central pain.

If, on the other hand, the hypothesis of Biemond (1956) that temperature-pain sensations are integrated at the level of the second sensory area is true, then clearly a lesion of the postcentral gyrus, which does not interrupt the spinothalamocortical paucisynaptic pain pathway at all, cannot possibly cause central pain. Moreover, if it is true that all the sensory areas (first, second, and supplementary) play a part in the integration of pain sensations, it is readily understandable that a circumscribed cortical lesion damaging only a tiny percentage of the pain fibers could not give rise to a sensory deficit or to central pain.

An exceptional case of spontaneous pain may throw some light on the problem. We refer to the case of Biemond (1956) (Fig. 19) that seems to show unequivocally that central pain from a cortical lesion presupposes interruption of the afferent fibers of the paucisynaptic system: a lesion of the second somatic sensory area gave rise to central pain and derangement of sensibility to temperature and pain without affecting epicritic sensibility.

There are thus several problems and they are not easy to solve. One point is, however, worth making: parietal cortectomy would seem to show that lesion of the pathways of epicritic sensibility is not an essential factor in the causation of central pain, for it is the epicritic sensibility system that is particularly affected at this level, as seems to be shown by the sensory disturbances caused by gyrectomy.

Petit-Dutaillis *et al.* (1950) declared that lobotomy, topectomy, and frontal lobectomy are consistently accompanied by obvious sensory disturbances in the first two months after operation and that they disappear completely with time. They take the form of trigeminal paresthesias, heightened reactions to pain and temperature stimuli, photophobia, and hallucinations and are thought to be due to liberation of the paleothalamus.

FIG. 19. Anatomicopathological findings in a case of central pain. The findings were areas of softening in the cortex of the parietal operculum and insula (dotted areas); retrograde degeneration of fibers coming from the posterior ventral nucleus of the thalamus, which cross the posterior portion of the capsula interna (shaded area); marked loss of cells in the VPM and VPL (striped area). The patient was suffering from severe hypoalgesia in association with continuous deep pain on the left side of the body. Tactile, deep, and stereognostic sensibility were intact. This case seems to show that for the onset of central pain from a cortical lesion injury to the pain pathways (third neuron of the paucisynaptic system) is sufficient without a concomitant lesion of the fibers of the epicritic system. *Source:* Constructed from the data of Biemond (1956).

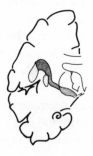

HEMISPHERECTOMY

Dandy (1933) in two cases of central tumor subjected to hemispherectomy observed hypoalgesia of the contralateral side of the face in one case and normal perception of pricking in the other; in the other body districts there was loss of all cutaneous sensations, but movements of the joints and compression of the muscles caused intense pain in both cases.

Bell and Karnosh (1949) observed "hyperpathia" of the limbs in cases treated by hemispherectomy; the phenomenon is transient, but even when it has completely subsided there remains a trace, that is to say, patients dread the application of any stimulus on the paralyzed side.

Obrador (1956) made similar observations.

Laine *et al.* (1952) and Laine and Gros (1956) pointed out that hemispherectomy may be followed by hyperpathic disturbances: all stimuli are perceived with a painful "tonality"; passive movement of the joints enhances the hyperpathia. According to these workers, these phenomena gradually pass off within a week or more.

Quarti and Terzian (1954) reported painful hyperesthesia of the limbs on the treated side in all their six cases. It lasted for about two weeks and it was thought to be due to thalamic irritation caused by coagulation.

Gardner *et al.* (1955) reported on a follow-up study they had made of patients subjected to operation for hemispheric glioma. Pain stimuli were felt with a "disagreeable" tone on the operated side; hot and cold stimuli were not felt as such but as pain stimuli. The authors did not state exactly how long after operation they made these observations but it was certainly a long time since the patients had survived operation for 1 to 17 years.

Zülch (1960) in a study of 13 cases of hemispherectomy reported that pain with the typical characteristics of central pain appeared in the majority of the patients.

On the other hand, many case series have been reported in the literature in which central pain was not observed.

Discussion

It is very difficult to evaluate the role of hemispherectomy in the causation of central pain because this operation is generally performed in patients affected with long-standing brain disorders who already have sensory deficits and in whom the hemisphere presumed to be intact has often taken over vicarious functions. Furthermore, many of the patients so treated are feeble-minded and so the gathering of information is difficult.

It is emphasized that many workers have observed central pain only in the first few postoperative days and that the thalamus is certainly injured in the surgical maneuvers, which may act as an irritant and thus precipitate these pains.

There is no doubt that hemispherectomy is the only operation that totally abolishes all the cortical afferent fibers originating in the relay nuclei of the thalamus and so interrupts all the tertiary neurons of the spinothalamocortical paucisynaptic pathway concerned with the transmission of pain stimuli. After this operation the functions of the removed hemisphere may clearly be discharged vicariously by the contralateral hemisphere or by subcortical structures. Moreover, in the hemispherectomized individual pain impulses may, as happens normally, converge on the brainstem-thalamic polysynaptic systems. The material of Gardner et al. (1955) is highly interesting: their patients were adults suffering from brain tumors and in such patients the intact hemisphere can rarely discharge vicarious functions as it can in children with brain disease. Hence, in these cases hemispherectomy permanently interrupts the transmission of pain impulses along the paucisynaptic pathway at the level of the third neuron; however, large numbers of the impulses can reach the brainstem and thalamus via the polysynaptic systems, a situation which probably favors the onset of central pain. It is for this reason that central pain lasted so long in the patients of Gardner *et al.* (1955). In the cases of hemispherectomy for non-tumoral diseases of the brain, on the other hand, several alternative pathways are opened, and pain impulses probably travel as far as the cortex via homolateral pathways; thus, despite the operation, the

FIG. 20. Diagram of presumed physiopathological pattern in children suffering from cerebral disease subjected to hemispherectomy. It is known that even in normal children a number of spinothalamic fibers run from the subthalamic region to the posterior ventral nucleus of the opposite thalamus (e.g., some fibers of the left spinothalamic tract end in the right VPL). In children suffering from cerebral disease with major neonatal hemisphere lesions it is probable that this contingent of fibers assumes a vicarious function and becomes hypertrophic, as occurs in the motor system for the pyramidal pathway (Zülch, 1963) and that the contingent of paucisynaptic fibers bound for the damaged hemisphere is of little functional importance. The removal of the diseased hemisphere in children suffering from cerebral disease thus probably causes little further impairment. This may explain why the postoperative pains either disappear quickly or do not arise at all in these cases, whereas they persist in cases of hemispherectomy performed in subjects with hemisphere lesions acquired in adult life.

(a) Spinothalamic tract; (b) VPL nucleus of thalamus; (c) damaged hemisphere.

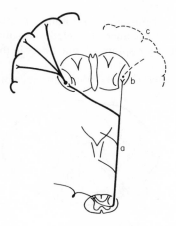

function of the paucisynaptic pathway is, in a sense, spared. This point may explain why in infantile hemiplegia hyperpathia does not always appear, and if it does, why it is usually short-lived (Fig. 20).

Naturally, hemispherectomy does not enable us to draw any conclusions regarding the importance of lesions of the epicritic systems in the genesis of central pain. But it is important to point out that in this operation, as in cortectomy, the polysynaptic systems and the reticular system of the brainstem and thalamus are spared. It would thus seem certain that lesion of the polysynaptic systems is not necessary for the onset of a central pain syndrome.

POSTERIOR CORDOTOMY (FIG. 21)

This operation has been performed both for pain syndromes and for spasticity. Pool (1946) treated three cases of phantom limb pain of the upper limb. He cut the posterior column of the spinal cord on the side homolateral to the pains (column of Burdach 3.5 mm deep) as well as the adjacent gelatinous substance of Rolando. The section was made at C5–C6. The author said that he obtained good results, which might have been due partly to the section of the posterior funiculi and partly to interruption

FIG. 21. Diagram of posterior cordotomy. The surgical lesion may extend to the tract of Lissauer, the gelatinous substance of Rolando, and probably even to the spinothalamic fibers in their course into the posterior horns.

(1) Tract of Lissauer; (2) gelatinous substance of Rolando.

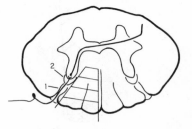

of the fibers of the gelatinous substance of Rolando, which transmit sensory impulses "different from the proprioceptive" ones, and also partly to interruption of the internuncial systems of the tract of Lissauer. The neurologic findings in the three cases are as follows:

CASE 1: Result on phantom limb pains incomplete. No motor or sensory disorders in the limbs. From the collarbone to the breast on the operated side the application of hot and cold stimuli to the skin produced an exaggerated unpleasant sensation of heat and cold. Pin-pricks in this area were not felt as sharply as in normal areas of the cutis and the patient reported a constant sensation of numbness and stiffness in this area, though this disappeared gradually within 8 weeks; there was no derangement of vibration sense or of tactile discrimination.

CASE 2: Result on phantom limb pains slight. The patient complained of the same sensations as in case 1 from the collarbone to the 11th rib. In addition, when he washed his face he felt a pulling sensation along the medial aspect of the phantom limb.

CASE 3: For 14 days after operation there was hyperesthesia over the left side of the thorax from the collarbone to D8; there was a deficit of vibration sense in the left foot and of sensibility to temperature and pain in S3–S5 on the right; these symptoms, which disappeared quickly, were put down to edema of the left half of the spinal cord.

Pool considered that the hypoalgesia and hyperthermoesthesia observed in all three cases at a distance from the level of the section were due not to lesions of the spinothalamic tract, which lies in the anterolateral quadrant of the opposite side, but to interruption of intersegmental sensory neurons on the same side, that is, of internuncial fibers in the tract of Lissauer.

Browder and Gallagher (1948) treated six cases of phantom limb pain by section of the posterior funiculi. Unlike Pool, they did not allude to the possibility that the substance of the posterior gray horns as well as the posterior funiculus may be cut during operation. They said that sensibility to light touch was unaffected by the operation; they reported no disturbances of sensibility to temperature and pain; in three cases there was some deficit of vibration sense and of position sense below the section. One patient complained of an intermittent burning pain on the amputation stump after operation, which apparently had not been there before; the authors did not comment on this. They did not report any central pain.

Grant and Weinberger (1941) attributed the paresthesias they had observed in limbs homolateral to the section after Siöqvist trigeminal tractotomy for trigeminal pains to the extension of the lesion to the homolateral cuneate nucleus.

White and Sweet (1955) stated that they had "never observed any significant neurological sequel from injury to the . . . nucleus cuneatus."

Pool (1946) and Browder and Gallagher (1948) are, as far as we know, the only workers to have used cordotomy of the posterior funiculi for treating pain syndromes, though this operation has been used often in cases of spastic paralysis.

Puusepp performed a 2.5-mm-deep section of the tract of Burdach in a patient suffering from postencephalitic parkinsonism; there was some loss of sensibility to light touch and a very slight derangement of deep sensibility.

Antonucci (1938) performed a bilateral section of the tracts of Goll in a patient suffering from Little's spastic paraplegia. The patient had normal sensibility to light touch, temperature, and pain; muscle and bone sensibility were not explored. The operation produced a distinct reduction of hypertonus. In the days following operation the patient complained of a feeling of numbness in one lower limb and for one night pain also, but by the 19th day these symptoms had completely disappeared.

Rizzatti (1939) performed a 4–5-mm-deep section of the tracts of Goll at the level of the tenth dorsal vertebra in a case of

Little's flexor paraplegia. The result on the spasticity was very good. Disturbances of sensibility could not be studied because the patient was mentally handicapped. No reference is made to central sensory phenomena.

Franceschelli and Clivio (1948) used Antonucci's method as modified by Zanoli in seven cases of spastic paralysis: instead of a cordotomy they performed 15–50 acupunctures into the posterior funiculi at thoracic level. The resulting disturbances of epicritic sensibility were slight. No central sensory phenomena were reported.

Feld and Pecker (1951) treated a case of extensor paraplegia by bilateral cordotomy affecting the inner two thirds of the posterior funiculi. They did not report any postoperative sensory disturbances.

Borellini (1948) reported on 13 cases of spastic paralysis of varied etiology treated with Zanoli's operation (15–50 acupunctures of the posterior funiculi); bilateral dorsal medial posterior cordotomy was performed in only one case. This worker reported that the sensory deficits consequent upon the Zanoli operation were very slight, whereas those consequent upon cordotomy were more marked. He did not report any central pain.

Bressan et al. (1956) in a paper that gave few precise details reported on the treatment of ten cases of spastic paralysis with acupuncture of the tracts of Goll and Burdach (according to Zanoli). In regard to sensory disturbances, they stated that only postoperative tactile hypesthesia could be elicited. They did not mention any central pain.

Discussion

The posterior cordotomy material involves a rather small number of operations, including some operations that were not strictly cordotomies; indeed the majority were acupunctures of the posterior funiculi. Further, many of the cases suffering from spastic syndromes were not studied thoroughly with regard to sensory phenomena.

The authors generally reported that alterations of sensibility, even of deep sensibility, were few after these operations on the posterior funiculi, but this may be due to the techniques employed. The only worker who, to our knowledge, explicitly quotes postoperative numbness and pain (even though the pain lasted only one night) is Antonucci (1938). According to the data of all the other workers it would seem that this operation does not produce true central pain. It would have been valuable to have larger case series and more precise information on the postoperative subjective sensory alterations: these would have supplied some useful indication as to the true role of the epicritic systems in the genesis of central pain in cord lesions.

The data supplied by Pool (1946), though very precise clinically, are difficult to interpret. He extended the lesion as far as the gelatinous substance of Rolando and hence inevitably to the tract of Lissauer that invests it; thus the true significance of the central symptoms that he clearly observed in his patients is difficult to assess. It should be noted, however, that the disturbances he observed had a girdle distribution on the side homolateral to the section. The band of dysesthesia was in one case narrow (probably only 3–4 dermatomes, case 1), whereas in the others it was broader (apparently 8–10 dermatomes).

It is interesting to compare these data with those of Hyndman (1942), who by cutting the tract of Lissauer produced a band of anesthesia to temperature and pain, associated in some cases with mild tactile hypesthesia and "subjective numbness" extending at least 4–5 dermatomes below the level of section. From the case records and from Hyndman's illustrations (Fig. 11) it would seem that the zone of anesthesia ensured by this operation actually extended in two cases from D1 right down to D7 and in one case from D4/5 to D11, that is, 6–7 dermatomes.

According to Hyndman (1942), these data show that the temperature-pain fibers of the tract of Lissauer and some of the tactile fibers may ascend as much as five segments before entering the posterior horns. Even he admitted, however, that some disturbances of tactile sensibility might be due to injury to the posterior funiculi.

It is clear that at least in case 1 of Pool, in which there were disturbances only of the temperature and pain sense, the dysesthesias could easily be explained by the interruption of ascending fibers in the tract of Lissauer. With regard to the other two cases, in which the temperature-pain dysesthesias and hyperesthesias extended several dermatomes below the level of section, always in a wide band, they were probably due to damage both to the tract of Lissauer (see Hyndman's data) and to the commissural fibers running from the posterior horns to the spinothalamic tract.

TRIGEMINAL TRACTOTOMY (SIÖQVIST'S OPERATION) (FIG. 22)

Rowbotham (1938) observed no facial dysesthesias after three of these operations.

Grant *et al.* (1940) treated 12 cases: four patients suffering from trigeminal neuralgia and eight from pain due to cancer. In all 12 cases hypoalgesia or analgesia was obtained in the facial territory and in eight cases tactile hypesthesia was observed. No paresthesias or central pain in the facial territory were reported.

Grant and Weinberger (1941) emphasized the importance of the level at which the incision in the bulb is made. If, as Siöqvist at first recommended, it is made 8–10 mm above the obex, the restiform body and the cuneate nucleus may be injured. Grant and Weinberger considered that injury to the cuneate nucleus was responsible for sensations of numbness in the homolateral half of the body that came on after operation in one of their patients; in one of Siöqvist's cases, on the other hand, the sensations of numbness were in the contralateral limbs. The authors stress that one of the advantages of Siöqvist's operation over posterior rhizotomy is that it does not injure the motor branch and

FIG. 22. Summary diagram of the trigeminal sensory pathway. Despite interruption of the descending root and of the sensory nucleus of V, pain impulses can obviously be diverted through the collaterals and the ascending branches of the bifurcated fibers onto the "intranuclear pathway" and onto the reticular formations of the brainstem, via which they reach the higher centers. This mechanism might explain the onset of central sensory phenomena after Siöqvist's tractotomy. Another mechanism that might explain the onset of central pain is as follows. The most caudal portion of the trigeminal nucleus probably receives impulses from the cervical roots or even impulses ascending through the polysynaptic system of the gelatinous substance of Rolando. Once the physiologic impulses of V have been eliminated by surgical section, the above impulses may "get the upper hand" in the "intranuclear pathway" of the trigeminal and so give rise to abnormal sensations. Very deep sections of the nucleus also interrupt the intranuclear pathway and probably prevent the onset of these abnormal sensations mediated by that pathway. The difference in depth of the bulbar section may explain why some workers have observed central sensory phenomena very frequently after Siöqvist's tractotomy and others very rarely.

(a) Nucleus oralis; (b) nucleus interpolaris; (c) nucleus caudalis,

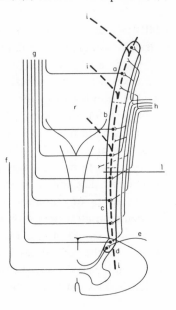

which receives all the pain fibers of V; (d) cervical region where the nucleus caudalis continues with the gelatinous substance of Rolando; (e) posterior cervical root; (f) spinothalamic tract; (g) quintothalamic tract; (h) sensory root of the trigeminal nerve; (i) "intranuclear pathway" (polysynaptic), which transmits impulses to the reticular formations of the brainstem; (r) reticular formations of the brainstem; (1) surgical section of the descending trigeminal root at obex level, which may involve the trigeminal sensory nucleus at a deep level.

---

leaves tactile sensibility unharmed and this is why, in their view, the face "does not feel cold and numb." They did not pursue the matter further: it would seem to be implicit in their line of reasoning that paresthesias from a central lesion are the consequence of injury to the systems of fibers of tactile and deep sensibility. It is pointed out, however, that they spoke only of numbness and of cold and not of pain.

Olivecrona (1947a and b) stated categorically that none of his 101 cases of trigeminal neuralgia treated with bulbar tractotomy complained of paresthesias or pain (painful anesthesia). On the other hand, one of 13 cases of migraine complained of postoperative paresthesia.

Le Beau et al. (1948) recorded no case of postoperative paresthesias or pains in a series of 20 patients who had suffered from facial neuralgia.

Grant (1948) observed paresthesias in two out of six cases.

Hamby et al. (1948) reported the follow-up findings in a series of 28 patients subjected to Siöqvist's tractotomy: 12 complained of facial dysesthesias, though less severe than those observed after trigeminal rhizotomy.

Falconer (1949) stated that all of his 20 patients complained of some disagreeable sensation in the analgesic area, often in the form of "pins-and-needles, tingling pains or itching sensations," but that none of them was unduly bothered by these sensations.

Guidetti (1950), reviewing the 124 cases of bulbar tractotomy for trigeminal neuralgia of Olivecrona, reported that eight patients complained of mild facial paresthesias but never so severe as those observed after trigeminal rhizotomy. It is rather odd that Olivecrona (1947a and b), writing about 101 of these 124 cases, never came across postoperative paresthesias.

Zülch and Schmid (1953) reported two cases (one bilateral): hyperpathia to deep pressure with summation phenomena for light touch appeared in the hypoalgesic facial territory in both cases.

White and Sweet (1955) observed a very high incidence of postoperative paresthesias and pains in the analgesic territory in a series of 32 cases treated with Siöqvist's operation: 18 for trigeminal neuralgia and 14 for facial pain from cancer. In two cases the paresthesias were reported to be unbearable, while in 18 others they were milder, and in some the patients only mentioned the fact if specifically questioned; in some cases the paresthesias were transient. These paresthesias usually come on about a week after operation or even later; they never come on immediately after operation; they may increase with time or diminish to the point of disappearing.

White (1962) stated that with tractotomy of the descending root of the trigeminal "the complication of facial paresthesia is not reduced" and so "a rather high proportion of subjects complain of unpleasant paresthesia afterwards."

Discussion

The onset of subjective sensory phenomena after tractotomy of the descending root of the trigeminal is a fairly frequent occurrence: about 30 percent of the cases in the material we have examined complained of these disturbances. The range of variation, however, is enormous: from Falconer (1949), who said that they were observed in 100 percent of cases, and White (1962), who held that they occurred in a high percentage of patients, to Olivecrona (1947) and Le Beau *et al.* (1948), who stated that they had never observed them. Probably the various workers take different views of the subjective phenomena reported by their patients. In any case, even those who report a high percentage of subjective sensory disturbances after operation say that they are often transient, usually in the nature of mild paresthesias, rarely like true pain and that they do not usually attain the intensity of the pains of painful anesthesia after Frazier's rhizotomy.

Siöqvist's operation consists in interruption of the descending root of V, usually at the level of the obex. Hence, from the physiopathological point of view the situation resulting from this operation is totally different from the situation arising out of retrogasserian rhizotomy despite the fact that both interventions interrupt the first sensory neuron. First, rhizotomy interrupts all the afferent fibers, while Siöqvist's operation interrupts only some of them. It is indeed known that the fibers of V bifurcate on entry to the pons, all of them according to some workers (Testut, 1943), only part according to others (Windle, 1926; Ranson and Clark, 1957; Peele, 1954).

According to Siöqvist (1938), the poorly myelinated fibers (under 4μ) transmitting pain impulses enter the descending root of V without bifurcating. It is therefore clear that a section at obex level spares all the ascending branches of the bifurcated fibers and many of the descending branches that terminate in the oral and interpolar portions of the trigeminal nucleus lying above the section. Only the fibers terminating in the caudal part of the nucleus, that is, the pain fibers, are interrupted.

Windle (1926) demonstrated that some fine descending fibers can give rise to collaterals and bifurcate once they have entered the neuraxis.

Furthermore, if it is true on the basis of Cajal's diagrams and the statement of Cajal (1899) and of Ranson and Clark (1957) that the ascending and descending fibers of the sensory tract of the trigeminal nerve give off collaterals which likewise end in the sensory nuclei and in the reticular formation, it is obvious that even if the pain impulses can no longer reach the cells of the caudal portion of the nucleus, from which the secondary fibers probably originate (quintothalamic tract: paucisynaptic pathway), they can still reach other cells of the sensory nucleus and the reticular formation via the spared collaterals. And as it is known that many cells of the sensory nucleus give rise also to short-axon fibers and that "they run in the reticular formation" (Ranson and Clark, 1957), as Stewart *et al.* (1964) have observed in the cat, it is highly probable that the pain impulses which can no longer reach the thalamus via the paucisynaptic pathway can still be transmitted by other systems of fibers, in all likelihood polysynaptic systems (Fig. 22).

Another point worth noting is that in the trigeminal nucleus there seems to be an ascending polysynaptic system originating, according to Stewart *et al.* (1964), in the caudal portion of the nucleus and rising to its rostral portion: this system transmits impulses to the reticular formations of the brainstem. This intranuclear polysynaptic pathway has in all probability a similar status to that of the supposed ascending polysynaptic pathway of the gelatinous substance of Rolando.

It is important to remember that the most caudal part of the descending nucleus of the trigeminal nerve receives impulses not only from nerves VII, IX, and X but also from the medial and lateral cuneate nuclei (Stewart *et al.,* 1963).

Moreover, according to Kerr (1961), the endings of the trigeminal and cervical primary neurons are superimposed in the upper reaches of the cervical cord, where the caudal portion of the trigeminal nucleus runs into the gelatinous substance of Rolando (Olszewski, 1950; Taren and Kahn, 1962). Hence the facial paresthesias and pains in the anesthetic territory after retrogasserian rhizotomy may well be due to activation of the caudal part of the trigeminal nucleus which transmits impulses of extratrigeminal origin to the higher centers via the "intranuclear pathway" (Stewart *et al.,* 1964). The same phenomenon can, we think, occur after Siöqvist's tractotomy if the section interrupts only the descending tract of the trigeminal nerve and not the nucleus with its "intranuclear pathway"; this is the second possible explanation of the onset of facial dysesthesias after Siöqvist's tractotomy. If, however, the incision interrupts the descending nucleus and its "intranuclear pathway," impulses ascending in this system may be blocked also; the occurrence of dysesthesias is thus more unlikely.

The different depth of the surgical lesion may perhaps explain why some workers have observed a high incidence of subjective sensory phenomena after Siöqvist's operation and others none. It should be remembered that in this operation the subjective sensory phenomena are due to lesion of the first neuron and that there is an anatomical substrate similar to that which is probably responsible for certain sensory phenomena resulting from damage to the first sensory neuron at spinal cord level.

PYRAMIDOTOMY AND EXTRAPYRAMIDOTOMY

OF THE SPINAL CORD

Putnam (1940) proposed section of the lateral pyramidal tract for parkinsonism (Fig. 23a). In commenting on his cases he did not mention any sensory deficits, though some of the case records refer to contralateral hypoalgesia. There is, however, no mention at all of central pain or dysesthesias.

Oliver (1949) reported on the results obtained in 48 cases of parkinsonism with lateral pyramidotomy. In the first group of patients the cut was only 4 mm into the cord; because the results were unsatisfactory it was decided to make the cut about 5 mm deep. The lesion was thus larger and sometimes impinged on the spinothalamic tract, in consequence of which patches of altered sensibility to temperature and pain appeared on the contralateral half of the body. No clinical signs of damage to the posterior funiculi were ever observed. There is no reference to central pain.

Oliver (1950) reported on the results obtained in cases of parkinsonism from an operation in which the lateral columns of

FIG. 23. Diagrams illustrating the operations of (a) Putnam: lateral pyramidotomy; (b) Oliver: extended lateral pyramidotomy; (c) Ebin: combined lateral and ventral pyramidotomy; (d) Putnam: anterior extrapyramidotomy; (e) Schürmann: combined pyramido-extrapyramidotomy. Although the lesion may extend to the pain pathways of the anterolateral funiculus in all these operations, central pains have been observed only in patients treated with the techniques of Oliver (b) and Ebin (c). With Oliver's operation (b), which involves complete section also of the spinothalamic tract of the anterolateral funiculus, central pains have been produced in the contralateral half of the body below the level of section. In all the other operations (a, c, d, e) the lesion of the spinothalamic tract is usually partial and the sensory deficit that may occur is generally slight and transient; Oliver's operation (b) results systematically in thermoanalgesia of the contralateral half of the body. The operations of Ebin (c) and of Schürmann (e) may involve injury to the posterior horns and the tract of Lissauer. Only Ebin (1949), however, reports "frequent" girdle pains homolat-

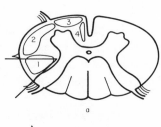

a

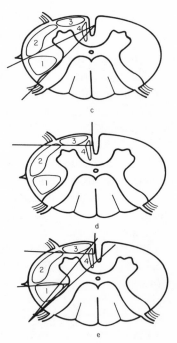

c

d

e

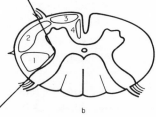

b

eral to the section attributable to lesion of the first neuron within the cord. It should be remembered that all these operations also involve more or less extensive interruption of the propriospinal polysynaptic systems.

---

the cord were completely cut at cervical level; hence the spinothalamic tract was cut as well as the pyramidal tract. This operation also causes permanent contralateral hemianalgesia; because the posterior funiculi are spared there is no derangement of epicritic sensibility. In one of his cases Oliver reported unpleasant "electric shock" type sensations in the leg on the side contralateral to the operation (Fig. 23b).

Ebin (1949) proposed a combined tractotomy designed to destroy the lateral and anterior pyramidal fibers simultaneously (Fig. 23c). This operation results in damage to the gray substance of the posterior and of the anterior horns, to the homolateral tracts of Goll and Burdach, and to the homolateral spinothalamic tract, although not extensively. In most of the 11 cases so treated, anesthesia to temperature and pain appeared in the contralateral leg, in some cases over a wider field, in some cases permanent, in others not. Ebin stated that he had often observed pains in the shoulder homolateral to the operation lasting several days or even months. Because the pain appeared in spite of every effort to spare the posterior roots of the cord, he thought that it must have been the consequence of damage to the fibers of the posterior roots within the cord or of damage to the gray substance of the cord.

Putnam (1933, 1938) reported in 1933 on the first results obtained in five patients suffering from extrapyramidal syndromes treated with anterior extrapyramidotomy (Fig. 23d). In no case did central pain appear, although in one case hypoalgesia and in another hemihypoalgesia were observed. The author did not discuss this sensory deficit. In 1938 he specified the pathways that were affected by this operation: vestibulospinal, tectospinal, and reticulospinal fibers extensively intermingled. In the first operations the incision was intended to include the rubrospinal tract also but the practice was abandoned because of the risk of injury to the pyramidal tract without any improvement in the result. Putnam also stated that if the lesion is too large it is likely to cause contralateral hemianalgesia. He mentioned no central pain or related phenomena in any of his 23 cases.

Schürmann (1953) reported on 33 cases of extrapyramidal affections and of spastic paraparesis treated with Putnam's anterior extrapyramidotomy. He made no reference to sensory disturbances or central pain in any of these cases.

Schürmann (1957) proposed a spinal cord operation for treating choreoathetoid syndromes: extensive section of half the cord including white and gray substances but sparing the tracts of Goll and Burdach. This operation of necessity causes deficit of sensibility to temperature and pain on the side of the body contralateral to the section and in some cases also deficit of epicritic sensibility. This worker records no central pain (Fig. 23e).

Discussion

The onset of central sensory phenomena after pyramidotomy and extrapyramidotomy is rarely mentioned. In some operations (lateral pyramidotomy and anterior extrapyramidotomy) the spinothalamic tract is theoretically spared, whereas in others the damage is not extensive (Ebin's combined pyramidotomy); in still others, section of the anterolateral funiculus and of the spinothalamic tract is inevitable (Oliver's and Schürmann's operations).

It is rather interesting that none of these workers described central sensory phenomena, with the exception of Oliver, who observed them in one of his cases subjected to hemisection of the cord, in which total section of the spinothalamic tract (anterolateral funiculus) is inevitable. The statistics are based on too few cases to be conclusive.

PHYSIOPATHOLOGICAL THEORIES ADVANCED TO

EXPLAIN THE ONSET OF CENTRAL PAIN

Many theories have been advanced to account for the onset of pain following lesions of the central nervous system, nearly all based on anatomicoclinical data for spontaneous damage. Although ingenious, many of these theories rest on conjecture rather than on sure physiopathological foundations.

It is only recently that some workers have tried to elucidate the physiopathological mechanisms of central pain and related phenomena by means of experimental research (Spiegel *et al.*, 1954; Poggio and Mountcastle, 1960) or by the anatomicoclinical study of central pain after surgery (Drake and MacKenzie, 1959; Mikula, 1959; Bowsher, 1959).

Many theories have been suggested to account for pains from thalamic lesions (Déjerine and Roussy, 1906; Roussy, 1907; Head and Holmes, 1911; Lhermitte, 1933; Noica and Balls, 1935) and a few to explain pain from lesions at any level of the neuraxis.

Very few workers have questioned whether spontaneous and induced sensory phenomena are mediated by the same physiopathological mechanisms and whether or not the various subjective sensations of which the patient complains, for example, paresthesias or pain, have the same physiopathological meaning (Sokolianski and Kulkova, 1938; Walker, 1955). Most workers have been concerned to establish which lesions of the nervous system were accompanied by altered or abnormally painful sensations and not to distinguish between spontaneous and induced phenomena or between true pain and other subjective sensations. Many theories have been put forward, but there are certain resemblances between them. We shall try to group them according to their physiopathological premises and see which are still tenable in the light of current knowledge of the physiopathology of the sensory systems, and whether the surgical data considered in some detail in the preceding chapters point to one rather than another type of theory.

THEORIES ATTRIBUTING CENTRAL PAIN TO IRRITATION OF THE SENSORY PATHWAYS OR CENTERS

Déjerine and Roussy (1906) described the anatomical lesion in three cases of thalamic syndrome and stated that the pains were due to destruction and "irritation" of the sense fibers arborizing in the ventral portion of the optic thalamus.

Nicolesco (1924) maintained that central pain is due to irritation of the nerve cells at the level of the sensory ganglia or of the relay nuclei of the spinal cord, bulb, and thalamus. He did not believe that irritation of the cortical neurons causes pain.

Garcin (1937) pointed out that even given lesions of the same site and size, central pains appear only in some patients and not in others. This is due to the anatomical characteristics of the tissue reaction to the lesion which, according to him, vary from individual to individual. He considered that irritation provided the most tenable theory of central pain: the irritated focus of the lesion is constantly bombarded by subliminal impulses from the periphery which under normal conditions are not felt but which are felt when the focus is irritated; the continuous transmission of the impulses explains the continuity of the pain.

He wondered whether a general theory could account for all types of pain; he thought that perhaps the pathogenetic mechanisms underlying pain from injury to the pain pathways might be different from those underlying pain from injury to the central receiving organ (thalamus).

Riddoch and Critchley (1937) and Riddoch (1938) thought that in cases of acute or subacute lesions that do not completely destroy the pain pathways phenomena which irritate nerve fibers and cells might be a factor in the causation of certain central pains.

THEORIES ATTRIBUTING CENTRAL PAIN TO AN ALTERATION OF THE FUNCTIONAL RELATIONS BETWEEN THE SYSTEMS CONCERNED WITH THE ELABORATION OF SENSORY PHENOMENA

According to these theories, among the various systems concerned with the elaboration of sensory phenomena there is one which regulates, dampens, or inhibits the functions of the others. Some workers think that this function devolves on the corticothalamic fibers; others think it is the paucisynaptic system of sensibility to pain; and still others, the epicritic sensibility system. Injury to this regulatory system results in a phenomenon of "liberation," which upsets functional balance and produces pain and related sensory phenomena.

Head and Holmes (1911) flatly rejected the irritation mechanism. According to them, central sensory phenomena are due to release of the thalamus from the restraining influence which the cerebral cortex exerts through corticothalamic fibers ending in the lateral region of the thalamus, where lesions responsible for the thalamic syndrome are usually found. Thus the cortex controls thalamic activity and injuries to these corticothalamic fibers result in hyperactivity of the thalamus. Hence, every afferent impulse capable of exciting the thalamus evokes exaggerated responses and sensations.

Riddoch and Critchley (1937) and Riddoch (1938) thought that central pain is mediated by several mechanisms depending on whether it is caused by incompletely destructive acute or subacute lesions or stabilized chronic lesions. In the former case irritative mechanisms play a part, but the fundamental mechanism of central pain is disintegration of the physiological processes underlying sensory activity. The main factor seems to be the reduction or loss of the damping mechanisms to which pain impulses are normally subjected. According to these workers, there is normally a process of integration of sensory impulses of all types; this process may occur at synaptic level or at any level of the neuraxis. In other words, a sensory impulse on arrival at the posterior horns undergoes a process of facilitation or inhibition through the action of different impulses of other origin; in its subsequent journey to the thalamus and cortex the impulse will be subjected at each synapse to the same processes of facilitation and inhibition. The impulses of epicritic sensibility (touch, position, pressure, and so forth) normally have a damping action on pain impulses, so when the impulses of epicritic sensibility are blocked they cease to exert this damping action and central pain appears. According to this theory, it is the physiologic pain impulses, heightened by the absence of restraint, that cause central pain. As the authors themselves indicated, this theory does not account for central pain in cases of complete analgesia, but as cases of central pain in analgesic subjects do occur, they supposed that the pain impulses are transmitted to the higher centers via pathways other than the spinothalamic tract. They considered that when strong stimulation is applied to the periphery the impulses may traverse the ipsilateral spinothalamic tract and perhaps also the posterior funiculi and the polysynaptic tracts of the gray substance of the cord (short relayed tract), according to suggestions by Foerster and others.

Frazier *et al.* (1937) believed that thalamic pain is the consequence of two factors: (1) an alteration at thalamic level of the afferent system of the posterior funiculi of the cord; indeed the epicritic system, in their view, exerts a damping action on the pain pathways; (2) a continual bombardment of temperature-pain impulses from the periphery, which in normal conditions might even be subliminal but which as a result of damage to the thalamus become supraliminal and give rise to central pain.

Kendall (1939) held that in the central nervous system there are two pain transmission systems: one slow and one fast. The two systems range over the whole neuraxis from the spinal cord through the brainstem to the thalamus. When a volley of impulses is triggered off by a pain stimulus, the impulses traveling in the fast, coarse fibers reach the central nervous system receptors before those traveling along the slow fibers; the latter impulses thus arrive late and find the receptors in "a relatively refractory state." Thus, in normal conditions the fast transmission system, which is thought to subserve the transmission of pain impulses with an epicritic component, inhibits at thalamic level the slow transmission system, which is thought to transmit protopathic pain sensations "with a high affective quality." Therefore, if there is an alteration of the fast system, the impulses conveyed by the slow system reach the receptors when they are not in a relatively refractory state; there is an exaggerated response to stimuli, which means a heightening of the pain sensation. According to this theory, central pain is due to injury to the fast pain fibers, which may be located at any level of the neuraxis from the cord to the thalamus and which spares the slow fibers.

Noordenbos (1959) expounded a similar theory, according to which there are two systems of pain impulse transmission: a fast one, that is, the spinothalamic tract and a slow multisynaptic system made up of the short-axon neurons of the gray substance of the cord. The multisynaptic system (MAS = multisynaptic ascending system) is similar to the reticular systems of the brainstem and would normally be under the inhibitory control of the fast transmission system, but when the fast fibers are damaged the inhibition no longer operates. Normally, impulses ascending the MAS are inhibited at every level of the cord by the fast transmission system through the action of impulses reaching the MAS via collaterals of the long fibers of the spinothalamic tract or through the action of impulses coming from the periphery via the fast fibers of the posterior root of the corresponding dermatome. Thus, as a result of any injury to the fast transmission system the inhibitory action exerted on the MAS becomes inadequate. Impulses ascending the MAS, on reaching the level of the injury, no longer sufficiently damped, cause pain which is referred also to distant dermatomes below the level of the injury. "Pain will occur, and this pain will be localized in the hyperaesthetic area. This pain is not caused by stimuli in that dermatome but occurs in absence of local stimulation. It is due to the action of the MAS, which represents nervous activity resulting from stimuli elsewhere."

Hassler (1960), like other modern workers, held that pain stimuli are conveyed both through the spinothalamic system and through the reticular systems of brainstem and thalamus. According to him, the reticular systems of the brainstem and thalamus, with a polysynaptic organization, are subject to the damping influence of the corticopetal systems concerned in the mechanisms of pain, which not only have a very low threshold but help to mitigate the distressing character of pain. Hassler considered that thalamic pain originates in the reticular systems, which he called the "trunko-thalamische System," because of destruction of the corticopetal systems, whose fibers originate in the nucleus caudalis (VPL) and nucleus ventrocaudalis parvicellularis (VCPC), the arrival point of the spinothalamic tract fibers.

Poggio and Mountcastle (1960) are, together with Spiegel *et al.* (1954), the only workers who have formulated a theory of central pain based on experimental data. They started from the observation that in apes a nociceptive cutaneous stimulus probably transmitted along the anterolateral funiculi (spinothalamic pathway) can activate cells of the postcentral gyrus and that these cells can be inhibited by stimuli conveyed by the epicritic sensibility system (medial lemniscus), that is, light touch stimuli applied to exactly the same point on the skin on which nociceptive stimulation had activated the cortical cells. Injury to the medial lemniscus might abolish this inhibitory activity. Hence, central pain would be due to release of the nociceptive system, which might be intact anatomically but no longer damped, as it usually is, by the lemniscal system of epicritic sensibility.

As we have seen, all the theories belonging to this group start from the assumption that central pain is caused by loss of a damping, restraining, or inhibiting function of a neuronal system put out of action by injury. Some other recent theories, such as those of Drake and MacKenzie (1953), Walker (1955), and Bowsher (1959), could, we feel, be included in this group, although these workers did not specifically mention such concepts as release from or abolition of damping mechanisms. They did, however, consider that central pain is due to injury to the spinothalamic system, the paucisynaptic pain pathway, which is put out of action; as a result the "spinoreticulothalamic" system (Bowsher, 1957), a phylogenetically older, polysynaptic system subserving the transmission of pain sensations that are ill-defined in time and place and unpleasant in quality, like central sensory phenomena, comes to the fore. As we have already seen, according to Noordenbos (1959) and Hassler (1960), the anatomical substrate for central pain and hyperpathia consists in these multisynaptic ascending systems in the spinal cord and brainstem (MAS according to Noordenbos and "trunko-thalamische System" according to Hassler). Let us now consider these concepts in greater detail.

Drake and MacKenzie (1953) held that central pain after mesencephalotomy is due to pain impulses conveyed in the reticular formations of the brainstem, via which they can still reach conscious level. This occurs when the spinothalamic tract is interrupted after it has given off collaterals to the reticular formation, as occurs in mesencephalotomy. According to these workers, the diffuse character of central pain and its late onset after the stimuli may be due to the fact that the impulses travel through a complex organization with a low speed of transmission, characteristics that are typical of systems with many synapses.

Walker (1955) held that the older theories explaining hyperpathia and thalamic pain in terms of release of the thalamus from cortical control are no longer tenable, because the lesions that give rise to thalamic pain interrupt the afferent fibers but do not isolate the thalamus from the cortex. Because these lesions interrupt the fibers afferent to the posterior ventral nuclear system of the thalamus to a greater extent than the fibers afferent to the nuclei of the mid-line, which belong to the reticular system, Walker believes that thalamic pain might be explained by the fact that after these lesions it is only or mainly the diffuse projection system of the thalamus, on which many pain fibers apparently converge, that remains active. This system has a low transmission speed, a diffuse cortical distribution, and is liable to give rise to "recruiting" phenomena; these physiological characteristics of the system might account for certain semeiologic characteristics of thalamic pain and hyperpathia. Walker wondered whether the pain fibers afferent to the nuclei of the thalamic reticular system might not be regarded as C fibers, like those of the peripheral nerves, which seem to be responsible for the onset of dysesthesias due to "fiber dissociation" mechanisms (Noordenbos, 1959) in lesions of the peripheral nerves involving the A fibers. Unless we have misunderstood Walker's line of reasoning, he considered that dissociation of the fiber spectrum such as that which occurs in peripheral nerve lesions might also underly thalamic pain.

Bowsher (1959) thought that the "spinoreticulothalamic" system is a link in the chain of neurons through which disagreeable, poorly localized pain sensations reach conscious level. This system closely resembles the activating reticular system of Moruzzi and Magoun (1949). Bowsher thought that massive cortical activation by impulses traveling along the reticulothalamo-cortical pathways of the diffuse projection systems may account for the onset of thalamic pain.

At this point we should mention the view of Mikula et al. (1959), which is completely opposed to the theories thus far quoted, regarding the possible participation of the reticular system in the pathogenesis of central pain. Mikula et al. (1959), on the basis of 25 spinothalamic tractotomies at midbrain level, maintained that the quantitative alterations suffered by the short

100

tracts of the reticular formation are of great importance: "plus l'incision épargne ce système [that is, the reticular] moindres sont les dysesthésies ultérieures." In the cases they operated on, dysesthesias appeared whenever the incision reached the medial planes of the midbrain and did not appear when the reticular system was spared. They considered that the disappearance of dysesthesias after a variable period could be explained by the operation of compensating mechanisms in the reticular substance.

THEORIES ATTRIBUTING CENTRAL PAIN TO LOSS OF A SPECIFIC THALAMIC FUNCTION

These theories seek to identify the origin of pain resulting from thalamic lesions. Most of them are based on the premise that the thalamus normally exerts a pain-moderating function.

Bonhoeffer (1928) considered that the thalamus has such a function, which is lost in certain lesions. Thalamic pain is thus the expression of diminished thalamic function.

Lhermitte (1933), contesting the theory of Head and Holmes (1911) (that thalamic pain is due to the release of the thalamus from cortical control) in cases of massive thalamic lesion, suggested another interpretation. The optic thalamus, which receives both superficial and deep stimuli, is to be regarded as an "analyzer," a "selective filter" of currents of general sensibility. It receives sensory impulses, transforms them in its synapses, filters them, arresting some and letting through others, which thus reach the cerebral cortex, where further discrimination is exercised. If this analyzing apparatus is only partially destroyed the sensory cortex receives coarse ("grossières") excitations that are normally stopped by the thalamus. Hence it is not the release of the thalamus that gives pain its affective color but injury to the analyzer apparatus of the organ.

Noica and Balls (1935) held that the thalamus exerts an automatic damping action on the stimuli that give rise to disagreeable and distressing pain. They based their conclusion on the observation that in some patients with a thalamic lesion agreeable sensory stimuli are perceived as such and not as pain even if applied to the side of the body affected by the thalamic syndrome, whereas disagreeable sensory stimuli cause pains typical of the thalamic syndrome. This moderating function of the thalamus is exerted, they thought, through a supposed "thalamic sympathetic system."

Rowbotham (1961) reported a case of intractable pain on the left side of face and skull in which histologic study disclosed lesions of the center median and ventroposterior lateral nuclei on both sides but more marked on the right side. He thought that the pains might be due to "misinterpretation of normal sensory messages at the thalamic level." This misinterpretation might be the result of altered function of the center median nucleus, which is a center that integrates the activity of the other thalamic nuclei. The fact that the pain was circumscribed to a small unilateral territory might, according to this worker, be explained more easily in neurophysiologic than in neuroanatomical terms. His suggestion is: "Possibly higher brain levels cannot interpret or misinterpret all the messages that come in at one time and may give precedence to messages that come along that pathway which at that time happens to be dominant."

We include in this group the hypothesis put forward by Walker (1955) to explain paresthetic phenomena. According to him, paresthesias from thalamic or subthalamic lesion are due to loss of an integrating function of the thalamus but he invokes another hypothesis to account for hyperpathia and central pain, as we have seen.

Walker (1955) considered that the thalamus has an integrating function in the process of elaboration of sensations, that is, it integrates the impulses that come in with several spatial and temporal characteristics (it is indeed well known that the impulses reaching the thalamus have some degree of somatotopic organization but are scattered in time because of the different transmission speeds of the fibers). The integration of impulses into "sensations" occurs normally only if they reach the posterior ventral nucleus with an appropriate "temporal" sequence. If the pathways afferent to this nucleus are injured, either at subthalamic or at thalamic level, the temporal sequence of the impulses is upset and the impulses are wrongly integrated, with resulting paresthesia.

THEORIES ATTRIBUTING CENTRAL PAIN TO IRRITATIVE IMPAIRMENT OF THE SYMPATHETIC SYSTEM

As far as we know, only Alajouanine *et al.* (1935) have ever specifically asserted that central pain may be due to irritation of the pathways or centers of the sympathetic system, though many workers have thought, largely on the ground that vasomotor and trophic disorders are often associated with central sensory phenomena, that the sympathetic system may play a part in the precipitation of pain even if the mechanisms invoked are not always clear.

Alajouanine *et al.* (1935) pointed out that central pains are as a rule accompanied by objective sensory disturbances, which are the result of destruction of the cerebrospinal pathways of sensibility. They therefore considered it a paradox to say that central pains were caused by irritation of sensory fibers or cells, since the destruction of the sensory pathways has no effect whatever upon these pains. These workers thought that underlying spontaneous pains and hyperpathia were a concomitant injury to the sympathetic system and stated that apart from the cerebrospinal system only the sympathetic system could transmit pain impulses and that there was no objection to the concept of a sympathetic origin for pain. This view is based on the observation that in central pain sympathetic disturbances (vasomotor, trophic, and sudoral) are the rule and on the assumption that there are sympathetic elements at every level of the sensory pathways. The sym-

103

pathetic system possesses a sensibility of its own, as shown by the fact that in patients operated on in spinal anesthesia, which suppresses cerebrospinal sensibility, irritation of the lumbar sympathetic chain precipitates pain reactions. The phenomenon of painful anesthesia would thus be easily accounted for: anesthesia is the expression of the destruction of the cerebrospinal sensory fibers and hyperalgesia is due to irritation of the sympathetic sensory fibers.

Garcin (1937, 1957) held that it was impossible to specify the role of the sympathetic system in the genesis of central pain. Sympathetic disturbances are neither a necessary nor sufficient condition of central pain; in fact, the vasomotor and secretory disorders observed in certain cases may be only reflex phenomena induced by pain.

Schuster thought that the medial nuclei of the thalamus might have a vegetative function; the fact that they are frequently involved in central pain syndromes raises the question, in his view, of whether they play a part in the genesis of central pain.

Pierre Marie (quoted by Garcin, 1937) thought that the sympathetic system doubtless played an important part in the production of thalamic pains.

Greiff (quoted by Garcin, 1937) attributed hyperesthesia to sympathetic vasomotor disturbances.

Ajuraguerra (1937) considered that the sympathetic system played an important part in the genesis of central pain. Actually it is not clear to us, despite the following explanation, quoted in full, how in the author's line of reasoning the sympathetic system can play a part in the causation of central sensory phenomena: "Nous croyons, cependant, que le sympathique joue un rôle, soit quand les algies produisent un retentissement sur le sympathique central ou même par voie indirecte par les modifications péripheriques produites par l'algie. Son action serait de modifier les douleurs, d'intervenir dans les variétés de celles-ci et dans leur déclenchement, mais non point d'en être toujours la seule cause."

THEORIES ATTRIBUTING CENTRAL PAIN
TO A MULTIPLICITY OF FACTORS

Some of the workers whose ideas we have outlined in the previous pages, while attributing key importance to a given mechanism, have considered that, at least in certain conditions, several physiopathological mechanisms might be involved. Garcin (1937), as we have seen, thought that the most important factor was irritation but that the altered functional relations between the various sensory systems might also play an important part. Ajuraguerra (1937) shared the views of Foerster (1927) but, as we have seen, also attached importance to the participation of the sympathetic system. Riddoch (1938) and Riddoch and Critchley (1937) attributed central pain to release phenomena but thought that irritation of the sensory pathways might be of importance in acute lesions. Wilson (1927) thought that dysesthesias (touch / pain / temperature complex) may be due to irritation of the afferent pathways and to release phenomena; but that on occasion sympathetic and vascular components may play an important part.

Foerster (1927) considered that there are two components in the genesis of central pain: irritation and release, that is, irritation of the pain pathways resulting from the lesion and release of the pain system from the damping mechanism that normally keeps it in check, so that all pain stimuli are freely transmitted. According to Foerster, the inhibiting activity is exerted by two systems: one is the system of epicritic sensibility, a phylogenetically recent system, and the other is a corticofugal system that makes itself felt at every level of the nervous system. He thought, moreover, that the striated system exerts an inhibiting action on the thalamus.

OTHER THEORIES

Theories on quite different lines have been advanced more recently by Zülch and Schmid (1953) and by Spiegel *et al.* (1954).

Zülch and Schmid (1953) and Zülch (1960) held that if one tries to find a common denominator for all cases of "hyperpathia" it can only be found in a numerical reduction of the functioning neuronal units ("numerischen Verringerung der funktionerenden Neuroneneinheiten") of the temperature and pain systems. After lesion of the sensory pathways hyperpathia occurs whenever the sensory substrate (that is, cells and fibers) "is so decimated numerically that for circumscribed pricking stimuli sensation can no longer come into being. For the diffuse stimuli of deep pressure the few units that are spared can still respond and this, through a summation phenomenon, results in the sensation of hyperpathic pain" ("Das empfindende Substrat ist . . . zahlenmäßig so dezimiert, daß auf den topisch umgrenzten Nadelstich eine Empfindung gar nicht mehr zustande kommen kann. Auf den diffus breitflächig ansetzenden Reiz des Tiefendrucks können die wenigen erhaltenen Elements aber noch ansprechen, was durch Summation zu dem . . . Ergebnis des hyperpatischen Schmerzes führt"). The authors adduced the example of hyperpathic phenomena localized on the side of the body opposite to that of the lesion consequent upon section of the spinothalamic tract at bulbar level resulting also in trigeminal hypesthesia. This means, in their view, that the incision extended too far back and spared part of the more ventral fibers of the spinothalamic tract. As further support for their hypothesis, these workers cited examples of Siöqvist's trigeminal tractotomy, in which a too anterior incision led to hypoalgesia or analgesia in association with hyperpathia on the contralateral side of the body: in these cases the lesion, being too anterior, cut a part of the spinothalamic tract. They therefore felt that hyperpathia could be treated only by surgical methods which resulted in complete interruption of the spinothalamic pain pathways.

These workers then went on to explain spontaneous central pains: hyperpathia may also be induced by superficial cutaneous stimuli (touching, rubbing) and the summation of these stimuli, such as that caused by the rubbing of clothes, may bring on apparently spontaneous pains.

Spiegel *et al.* (1954) and Spiegel and Wycis (1962) in explaining pain from thalamic lesion start from the assumption that a conscious integration of pain sensation can occur also at hypothalamic level. Their hypothesis is based on experimental data. In cats destruction of the posterior ventral nucleus of the thalamus (a lesion similar to that which produced Déjerine and Roussy's syndrome in man) results in an increase of the potentials evoked by peripheral stimulation at hypothalamic level. According to these workers, this is due to the fact that the impulses which, as a result of the lesion, no longer reach the thalamic nuclei are "diverted to the hypothalamus via bypaths which are normally only accessory routes." This increase in the impact of pain impulses on the hypothalamus would explain thalamic pain and the emotional and vegetative components that often accompany it. In cases of small lesions of the posterior ventral nucleus, impulses are diverted not only towards the hypothalamus but also "along normally less used collaterals" toward groups of cells of the posterior ventral nucleus close to the lesion: this fact might explain the hyperpathia that may be observed in regions adjacent to hypesthetic areas. These workers observed experimentally that if lesions of the posterior portion of the thalamus were very extensive (and impinge, for example, "upon the cerebral peduncle") they might prevent diversion of the afferent impulses to the hypothalamus. This experimental datum might explain why thalamic hyperpathia may disappear after a new, larger lesion in the posterior ventral nucleus of the thalamus. Further data are then cited to account for other aspects of central pain. It is pointed out that when the parietal cortex is deprived of some of its afferent connections by damage to the posterior nucleus of the thalamus, it becomes hypersensitive to stimuli coming from the periphery and to drugs (for example, metrazol). These hypersensitivity phenomena may act as accessory mechanisms in the thalamic syndrome, assuming, of course, that the cortex plays a part in the integration of pain. Actually, for the authors the cortex is not essential for the genesis of hyperpathia; it may perhaps play a fundamental part only in cases in which the brain lesions extend to the white substance below the cortex.

CLINICAL FEATURES OF SENSORY

PHENOMENA CONSEQUENT UPON LESIONS

OF THE CENTRAL NERVOUS SYSTEM

PAIN AND PARESTHESIAS: SPONTANEOUS AND INDUCED PHENOMENA

The clinical features of central pain syndromes have been studied extensively from every point of view (Garcin, 1937; Ajuraguerra, 1937; Riddoch and Critchley, 1938). There is therefore no point in going over all this material again, especially as it is now clear from the extensive literature on the subject that the clinical syndrome is protean and that a lesion of the central nervous system can give rise to any subjective or objective sensory symptom.

A point that does need stressing is that the workers who have concerned themselves with this subject have often used the same term to designate different clinical features or several terms to designate the same feature when describing the symptomatology. Noordenbos (1959) devoted a whole chapter of his monograph to the problem of terminology, pointing out the confusion of terms that has grown up, resulting in part from the desire of some workers to invent specific terms for certain phenomena, for example, psychroesthesia (hyperesthesia to cold), alloparalgia, synaesthesalgia (accentuation of pain by stimuli of an emotional nature), and so on. All these terms simply point to an alteration of the relation between the stimulus and the sensation induced, and as Noordenbos (1959) says, the fact that they "designate a number of conditions or syndromes with varying overlap" further complicates the situation.

A further source of difficulty and confusion is our channel of information regarding subjective sensory phenomena: the patient himself, in whom many symptoms are often associated and overlap. We feel that a fairly simple and convenient way of classifying central sensory phenomena, even though purely clinical and very summary, is to group them as follows:

Spontaneous Phenomena. These comprise all sensory phenomena that the patient complains of, from mild paresthesias to severe pain, arising apparently spontaneously, that is, apparently unprovoked by peripheral stimuli. Actually many of these phenomena, perhaps all of them, are due to peripheral stimuli (exteroceptive or interoceptive) which the patient for the most part fails to notice, or if he does notice them, misinterprets.

Induced Phenomena. These comprise all sensory phenomena that arise as a result of sensory or psychic stimuli which evoke an "exaggerated" or "perverted" response, often characterized by a "painful," "disagreeable," or "unfamiliar" quality. The sensations may be perverted in one or more of their fundamental characteristics: intensity, duration, topographical distribution with respect to the area stimulated, time of onset after the stimulus, mode of onset, and the affective component. The threshold for the stimuli capable of provoking these phenomena may be lowered (hyperesthesia) or raised (as occurs in the hyperpathia of classic writers). All these phenomena may coexist in a given patient, and, of course, both spontaneous and induced phenomena may coexist.

As the term "hyperpathia" recurs often in the literature, we would recall Head's description of the phenomenon. Hyperpathia means a pain reaction to any sensory stimulus whatever characterized by explosive onset of the pain sensation; lack of proportion between the intensity of the stimulus and the intensity of the response, which is always the same, as if the response obeyed only the all-or-none law; an extremely unpleasant quality often accompanied by intense emotional reactions; late onset; long duration; poor localization and distribution extending often throughout one half of the body; raised threshold (according to Riddoch, 1938, the threshold of hyperpathia may be normal, raised, or lowered).

TOPOGRAPHY OF CENTRAL PAIN

A study of the clinical features in correlation with the site, size, and type of lesion may perhaps supply some interesting material for the physiopathological interpretation of central sensory phenomena. A study of sensory deficits accompanying them is also of interest because it may yield indications as to the sensory systems affected by the lesion. We dealt with part of this problem in the description of the pathological anatomy of spontaneous lesions and in the exposition of the data relating to central pain from surgical lesions.

In many cases in addition to derangement of general sensation there are symptoms which are attributable to injury to other systems (pyramidal and extrapyramidal, cerebellar, and so on); these accompanying symptoms often point to the level of the injury. Is it possible to diagnose the level of injury solely on the basis of the topography of the subjective sensory phenomena and could this datum supply clues to the pathogenesis? Because this is such an interesting question, we shall now cite the most pertinent data in the literature on the topography of subjective phenomena on the basis of the site of the lesion. The data will be set forth very succinctly with frequent reference to the works summarizing the subject: those of Garcin (1937), Ajuraguerra (1937), and others.

Topography of Pain from Spinal Cord Lesions. Garcin (1937) summed up the topographical features of these pains according to the site of the lesion as follows:

(a) pains from injury to the posterior horns are on the same side as the injury, derive from one or more roots, and correspond to the affected metameres of the spinal cord;

(b) pains from injury to the anterolateral funiculus are due to interruption of the spinothalamic tract and essentially affect the whole area below the lesion but on the opposite side of the body; in some cases the pains are confined to circumscribed areas but these are always below the lesion. This is due to the fact that the sensory fibers are arranged increasingly in layers in the upper reaches of the spinal cord;

(c) pains from injury to the posterior funiculi are on the same side as the injury. In hemisections of the cord pain is usually observed below the lesion on the same side (posterior funiculi!) often with a "hyperalgesic" character, "more rarely pain phenomena are on the side contralateral to the section" (spinothalamic tract!).

Discussion

Many of these data tally with those emerging from the study of surgical lesions.

Pains with a "root" distribution homolateral to the lesion are homolateral to the section and may perhaps be due to real injury to the roots but also to damage to the cells of the posterior horns or even to damage to the first neuron in its intramedullary course (see pp. 43 and 82–83).

Surgical experience confirms that pains from section of the anterolateral funiculus have a contralateral sublesion projection, that is, they radiate to the peripheral projection territories of the damaged fiber system. Of greater interest is the problem of pain from section of the posterior funiculi. Apart from the case of Antonucci (1938), surgical experience has not proved beyond doubt that pain can arise from lesion of the posterior funiculi. But it does seem to be demonstrated (Weinberger and Grant, 1941) that paresthesias may be due to this type of lesion. White and Sweet (1955), on the contrary, stated: "We have never observed significant neurological sequel from injury to the . . . nucleus cuneatus." Mansuy *et al.* (1944) and Wertheimer and Lecuire (1953) reported on very large case series of commissural myelotomies. They observed "dysesthesia" or "paresthesia" type disturbances in the lower limbs, but one cannot be sure of the origin of these because the data on the operating technique and the level of the cord sectioned are scanty. The paresthesias were probably due to injury to the fasciculus gracilis, because this operation involves splitting the posterior funiculi (p. 45). These workers do not mention pain in the lower limbs but they do mention root pains at the level of the section. It would be interesting to know whether the dysesthesias and paresthesias in the lower limbs were accompanied by derangement of the heat-pain sense in the large case series of Wertheimer and Lecuire (1953).

In concluding this discussion, it is interesting to recall the statement of Riddoch and Critchley (1937) to the effect that there is no case in the literature of a unilateral lesion of the spinal cord with bilateral projection of pain and hyperpathia.

Topography of Pain from Injury to the Bulb and Pons. All writers on this subject (Garcin, 1937; Ajuraguerra, 1937; Riddoch, 1938) are agreed that pains arising in bulbar lesions, normally due to occlusion of the inferior posterior cerebellar artery (Wallenberg's syndrome), usually have an alternating distribution: trigeminal pain on the lesion side and pains in the contralateral side of the body. All or part of one side of face and body may be affected by these pains and in some cases the facial pain is bilateral. In lesions of the pons the facial and body pains are usually confined to the side opposite to the lesion. But there have been cases of bulbopontine lesions that obey no rule (Ajuraguerra, 1937) in which the pains affected the lower limbs and one side of the face.

Discussion

Pains with an alternating distribution are easily explained if one assumes that the lesion impinged on the descending tract of the trigeminal nerve and on the spinothalamic tract lying immediately in front of it, because the former conveys impulses from the homolateral side of the face and the latter from the contralateral side of the body. Cases in which the pains have a projection that apparently does not comply with the anatomical schemes to which we are wont to refer have not always been explained. It is often difficult to account for these phenomena in spontaneous lesions because of the irregularity, poor demarcation, and extent of the lesions. Riddoch (1938) was the only one to tackle the problem, and he reached the conclusion that bilateral trigeminal pain in bulbopontine lesions is due either to simultaneous injury to the two descending roots of the trigeminal nerve or to injury to the descending root on one side and to the

FIG. 24. Diagram representing a bulbar lesion involving the descending root and the sensory nucleus of V on one side (a and b) and the quintothalamic (c) and spinothalamic (d) tracts from the contralateral side. This lesion may cause central pain in both trigeminal territories and in the side of the body contralateral to the lesion.

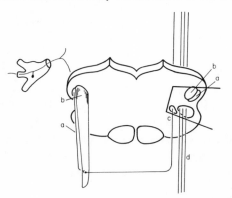

quintothalamic fibers coming from the other side which have already crossed the mid-line. Riddoch and Critchley (1937) said that bilateral central pain was impossible in unilateral lesions of the brainstem, except, of course, for trigeminal pain, because the pathways of this nerve have a peculiar distribution.

Surgical experience fully confirms these conclusions: the case of Zülch and Schmid (1953) (see pp. 51 and 106) is practically an experimental reproduction of these situations, and the data of Crawford and Knighton (1953) perfectly fit the hypothesis of Riddoch (1938) regarding bilateral trigeminal pains from injury to the descending tract and to the quintothalamic tract (Fig. 24).

In conclusion, the territory to which pains or dysesthesias are referred is the one tributary to the injured paucisynaptic system. The data for spontaneous lesions and those for surgical lesions fully agree on this point.

Topography of Pain from Injury to the Midbrain. As mentioned before, cases of central pain from spontaneous lesions at this level are exceptional (Noordenbos, 1959). The only data of help to us are the data for surgical lesions. Here again the distribution of pain follows the anatomical schemes: pains and paresthesias occur only in the side of the body contralateral to the section of the spinothalamic tract, which probably, at least in some cases, is isolated at this level without concomitant involvement of the lemniscal pathways.

Topography of Pain from Injury to the Thalamus. Garcin (1937) pointed out that pain due to thalamic damage has a hemiplegic distribution and affects the side of the body contralateral to the lesion, with a predilection for the extremities. Ajuraguerra (1937) stressed that the extent of the pain varies greatly: very often the whole of one side of the body is affected, sometimes only the face and upper limb, in rare cases the face only; moreover, in the course of the disease the pain may wander, disappearing from one limb only to arise in another. The sensory disturbances are likewise very variable: intense pains in the limbs may be found contemporaneously with only paresthesias in the face. Riddoch and Critchley (1937) pointed out that thalamic pain is usually found either throughout one side of the body or only in a small region: an arm, a leg, or the face on the side contralateral to the lesion, though cases of bilateral central pain resulting from unilateral lesions of the thalamus have been observed.

Garcin and Lapresle (1954) described a case of thalamic syndrome with pains in the hand and face on the side contralateral to the lesion, which was confined to the middle part of the VPL and to the lateral part of the VPM. Garcin (1937) reported cases of small lesions of the VPL thalamic nucleus with localized pains.

Discussion

Central pain from thalamic injury seems to depend upon the size of the damage to the VPL and VPM. The symptoms are more likely to be referred to the regions of the body which are thought to have most extensive representation at thalamic level (extremities of the limbs, for instance—Riddoch and Critchley, 1937) and, as we have seen, there have been cases in which pain had a somatotopic distribution corresponding to the size of the lesion (Garcin and Lapresle, 1954). We would recall that Riddoch and Critchley (1937) hypothecated a bilateral representation at thalamic level to explain the exceptional cases of bilateral pains from a unilateral lesion.

There are few cases in the literature of surgical lesions of the thalamus followed by central pain and these are not adequately backed by anatomicopathological evidence.

We have observed central pain in seven out of 24 cases treated with stereotactic operations on the sensory nuclei (VPL, VPM). Necropsy was done in cases 1 and 2 (see Appendix). The lesions affected a large part of the posterior portion of the thalamus, impinging to a greater or lesser degree on the VPL, VPM, and CM nuclei, the diffuse projection structures of the lamina medullaris interna and the LP and DM nuclei. In case 1 the pains affected a circumscribed territory: one side of the face and chest and one upper limb, although the anatomical lesion probably involved the entire VPL and there were serious sensory deficits throughout one half of the body. In case 2 central pain affected all of one side of the body and the lesion totally destroyed the VPL and VPM, extending quite a distance upward. In the other five cases (3, 4, 5, 6, and 7), in which there is no necropsy evidence, the pain affected the whole of one side of the body (4, 5) or was localized in a few areas (case 7, face and upper limb only).

The study of thalamic lesions would seem to show that destruction of the sensory relay nuclei (VPL and VPM) are necessary for the onset of central sensory phenomena and that the topography of the pain corresponds to the somatotopic representation destroyed by the thalamic lesion.

This point seems to be borne out by the stereotactic surgery evidence: central pain appears only in cases of damage centering on the sensory nuclei. To our knowledge, central pain has never been reported after the thousands of operations that have been carried out all over the world for lesions of the anterior, dorsomedian, lateroposterior, and ventrolateral nuclei. It is interesting that, on the surgical evidence, damage to the diffuse projection system of the thalamus, which is very often injured at the level of the reticular nucleus when coagulating the ventrolateral nucleus, does not give rise to central pain.

Unfortunately, our sketchy knowledge of the way in which the pain fibers end in the thalamus, the likelihood of their mixing with the epicritic sensibility fibers, the extent of the lesions (such that a "pure" lesion of the parvicellular ventrocaudal nucleus of Hassler —regarded by some as the pain relay center —is a quasi-impossibility), and the consistent simultaneous damage to the epicritic systems make it impossible for us to say, on the basis of thalamic lesions, whether the pain is the consequence of damage to the pain pathways only, as would seem to be demonstrated at midbrain, bulbar, and spinal levels, or whether simultaneous damage to the epicritic pathways is necessary.

Topography of Pain from Injury to the Cortex. Many workers consider that such pains exist. Riddoch and Critchley (1937) thought that pains and disagreeable sensations due to a cortical lesion are referred as a rule to the distal parts, face, hands, and feet, that is, to regions which seem to have most extensive cortical representation.

Discussion

As far as we know, central pain has not been described after surgical removal of the parietal cortex.

To conclude, central sensory phenomena, whether simple paresthesias or true pains, are referred topographically to the territory of the sensory system affected. But the site of a lesion can be diagnosed on the basis of the subjective central sensory phenomena in two conditions only: (1) in lesions of the posterior gray horns at spinal cord level or of the fibers of the first neuron in its intramedullary course when these lesions give rise to sensory phenomena with a fixed, constant, and definitely radicular distribution; (2) in lesions at bulbopontine level, which give rise to an alternate sensory syndrome.

TIME OF ONSET AND DURATION OF CENTRAL SENSORY PHENOMENA

It seems possible that a study of the time of onset of central sensory phenomena and of their duration might throw some light on the physiopathogenesis of these pains.

Immediate onset might constitute an argument in favor of release mechanisms, while late onset might suggest irritation of fibers and cells by a scarring process. The clinical and surgical evidence shows, however, that the time of onset is exceedingly variable. And one must never forget the observation of Garcin (1937), which every surgeon can confirm, that given a lesion with the same characteristics, extent, and site, only some patients will present central pain, a fact which obviously compounds the problem. Garcin (1937) tried to get around the difficulty by suggesting that the individual tissue reaction at the level of the lesion must be one of the factors conditioning the onset of pain. We will now quote briefly the salient data from the literature on these problems.

In thalamic and bulbopontine syndromes from vascular lesions the pains may come on immediately after the ictus or later (Ajuraguerra, 1937; Garcin, 1937); in some cases the pains may actually precede the other neurologic disorders (Ajuraguerra, 1937; Garcin, 1937). Pain from cortical and suprathalamic subcortical vascular lesions likewise appears early, as a rule (Riddoch, 1938). Baudouin and Lhermitte (1932) tried to establish a correlation between the time of onset of the pains and the type of vascular lesion, and they considered that the onset was immediate in hemorrhage and later in softening of the brain.

The literature on central pain of surgical origin likewise shows that the time of onset in cases of lesions of the same site and extent and induced by the same procedure varies enormously: sometimes the pains come on during the first few days after operation (Dogliotti, 1938; Walker, 1942; Lapresle and Guiot, 1953; Drake and McKenzie, 1953) and sometimes not until several weeks or months later (Walker, 1942; Lapresle and Guiot, 1953; Drake and McKenzie, 1953; Mikula *et al.,* 1959; Hassler and Riechert, 1959; Brihaye and Rétif, 1961; White, 1963).

Our experience of stereotactic surgery at thalamic level provides similar material: in one of our cases (see Appendix, case 6) the pain appeared immediately after coagulation, in five cases (2,

3, 4, 5, 7) it appeared from 6 to 12 days after operation, in one (case 1) a month and a half later.

Whereas the subjective central sensory phenomena due to pathologic spinal cord lesions are fleeting and short-lived (Ajuraguerra, 1937, Garcin, 1937; Riddoch, 1938), those due to vascular lesions of the bulb, pons, or thalamus last for a long time and rarely disappear completely, though they may vary in the course of time in intensity and even in site (Ajuraguerra, 1937; Garcin, 1937; Déjerine and Roussy, 1906).

Pains and paresthesias of surgical origin, including those due to section of the spinal cord, are generally long-lived (months, years) and often last until death (Lapresle and Guiot, 1953; Brihaye and Rétif, 1961; Horrax and Lang, 1957; Roeder and Orthner, 1961).

In regard to paresthesias and pains from Siöqvist's trigeminal tractotomy and from lateral mesencephalotomy, White and Sweet (1955) and Wycis and Spiegel (1962) state that they are generally transient.

In our experience (see Appendix) of eight cases of central pain following stereotactic thalamotomy only one showed complete remission of pain after 15 days (case 3); in two cases the pain lasted until death 5 months (case 1) and 27 days (case 2) after operation; in five other patients still living the sensory disturbances continue 12 months (case 4), 3 months (case 5), 2 months (case 6), 5 months (case 7) and 16 months (case 8) after operation.

A study of the duration of the symptoms thus shows that in the majority of cases the pains are irreversible, as if a permanent new physiopathological equilibrium were established as a result of the lesion, in consequence of which sensations no longer reach conscious level as normal sensations but have an altered character and often an intensely painful overtone. Once this new functional equilibrium is established and the lesions have stabilized the situation remains unchanged: the pains persist and efforts to allay them are generally without avail.

SURGICAL TREATMENT OF CENTRAL PAIN

Ever since the first description by Déjerine and Roussy (1906) it has been known that medical therapy is ineffective against central pain.

We have searched the literature for case material on the surgery of central pain. It is emphasized that the operations are the same as those which, performed in other patients in order to allay pain, have sometimes given rise to central pain. There are few cases of surgery for central pain in the literature, and as far as we know, no work in which this material has been reviewed and an evaluation of the results attempted in the light of modern ideas on the pathogenesis of central pain. In our review we shall obviously not be concerned with macroscopic lesions of the neuraxis, in the main of the cortex, that can be treated with surgical removal of the lesion (growths, vascular malformations, and so on) and we shall confine ourselves to cases in which the central pain called for functional surgery of the pain pathways.

We have considered only central pain attributable with a high degree of probability to circumscribed lesions of the central nervous system excluding tabetic, postherpetic pains, and so on, and those peculiar pain syndromes in which the pain is said to be "centralized" but whose physiopathological mechanisms have not been elucidated, such as phantom limb pains.

As indicated later, the operations were performed only in cases of outright pain and not in cases of mild disorders — paresthesias — even though of central origin.

OPERATIONS ON THE ROOTS AND PERIPHERAL NERVES

Apart from one case (Frazier *et al.*, 1937), radicotomy has been performed only for central pain in the trigeminal region.

Garcin (1937) reported the following cases: Foix treated one case of central pain from syringobulbia by alcohol injection of the gasserian ganglion without obtaining any improvement. Foerster obtained no improvement in one case. Schaeffer abolished pains from syringobulbia by means of a Frazier retrogasserian neurotomy. Ravina and Haguenauer, and Parker obtained good results.

Frazier *et al.* (1937) treated a case of central pain after vascular hemiplegia extending to the whole of one side of the body (face included) with bilateral cordotomy, alcohol injection of the gasserian ganglion, and radicotomy of C2–C3, with good results. On the strength of this case they felt that the future treatment of central pain would be cordotomy, where necessary bilateral, in association with section of the trigeminal fibers.

Spiegel *et al.* (1952) reported a case of thalamic pain localized in the face in which trigeminal rhizotomy was completely unsuccessful, as were a subsequent cortectomy and a lobotomy. Beneficial results were obtained with stereotactic mesencephalotomy.

White and Sweet (1955) noted no improvement in a case of facial pain secondary to a thrombotic lesion of a vessel of the medulla oblongata either with alcohol injection of the third branch of the trigeminal or of the gasserian ganglion or with retrogasserian rhizotomy or with alcohol injection of the sympathetic system.

Rowbotham (1961) reported a case of intractable pain in the left side of the head and face in which necropsy disclosed cellular fallout in the center median nucleus and in the adjacent portion of the VPL of both thalami, though more severe on the right. Neither retrogasserian neurotomy nor stellectomy was at all efficacious.

Bonica (1954) stated that peripheral analgesic block may be attempted when for any reason no other surgical procedure is feasible. The theoretical principle underlying these blocks is as follows: they eliminate normal afferent stimuli which in a person suffering from central pain may be appreciated with a painful "tonality." He reported the case of a 59-year-old woman with thalamic pain of vascular origin who had been repeatedly treated with paravertebral pantocain blocks and who was later treated with subarachnoid alcohol. The result was good for two months; the pain returned but another subarachnoid alcohol block once again gave good results.

OPERATIONS ON THE SYMPATHETIC NERVE

Turnbull (1939) reported a case of thalamic pain in the hand and forearm which 8 years after onset was treated with sympathetic block but without effect.

Hécaen et al. (1949) reported that in one of their cases of thalamic pain syndrome following a thalamic vascular lesion attempts at sympathetic infiltration and stellectomy were unsuccessful.

White and Sweet (1955) (case reported on p. 122) injected alcohol into the right thoracic sympathetic for pain in the right side of the face in a patient who had already undergone alcohol injection of the third branch of the trigeminal and of the gasserian ganglion without improvement; the operation on the sympathetic nerve likewise proved valueless.

Rowbotham (1961) (case quoted on p. 122) in a case of craniofacial pain in which retrogasserian rhizotomy had brought no relief tried stellectomy, but this was also unsuccessful.

Campanini and De Risio (1962) reported a case of hemiplegia from brain disease of childhood with deranged sensibility and thalamic pains which were distinctly improved by stellectomy. They attributed the good result to the improved blood supply to the injured hemisphere.

OPERATIONS ON THE SPINAL CORD AND BULB (SPINOTHALAMIC TRACTOTOMY AT SPINAL CORD LEVEL—ANTEROLATERAL CORDOTOMY—AND AT BULBAR LEVEL)

Turnbull (1939) (case quoted on p. 123) reported immediate abolition of pain by anterolateral cordotomy at cervical level in a case of thalamic pain in the hand and forearm in which sympathetic block had brought no relief.

Frazier *et al.* (1937) (case quoted on p. 122) reported a case of thalamic pain arising after a vascular lesion in which they performed bilateral cordotomy and homolateral radicotomy of C2–C3, which completely controlled the pain on one side of the body; the facial pains had been treated by alcohol injection of the gasserian ganglion.

Stone (1950) obtained no improvement with cervical anterolateral cordotomy in a case of central pain in one arm resulting from a vascular lesion.

White and Sweet (1955) treated a typical thalamic syndrome with anterolateral cordotomy at C2: although the level of analgesia was very high, C3–C4, there was no relief from pain. A subsequent parietal gyrectomy gave a satisfactory result but only for a few months. The same authors reported another case: a patient subjected to thoracic cordotomy complained after the operation of electrical discharge sensations and of burning sensations precipitated by hot, cold, and pricking stimuli applied to the area below the cordotomy. A further cordotomy performed two segments higher abolished these disturbances.

Bohm (1960) reported a case of burning sensations in the lower limbs after bilateral thoracic cordotomy; the patient was subjected to a further bilateral cordotomy two segments below the previous one but the burning sensations remained.

Bonica (1954) stated that in pain syndromes from spinal cord lesions anterolateral cordotomy above the lesion responsible for the pain might be useful.

Drake and McKenzie (1953) performed an intramedullary tractotomy in a case of central pain after lateral mesencephalotomy; the pain disappeared altogether.

OPERATIONS ON THE MIDBRAIN (OPEN LATERAL MESENCEPHALOTOMY AND STEREOTACTIC MESENCEPHALOTOMY)

Walker (1942a) performed an open lateral mesencephalotomy on a case of thalamic pain; the patient died 26 hours later.

Roeder and Orthner (1961) performed a stereotactic coagulation in which the chief target was the reticular formation of the midbrain in a woman suffering from postapoplectic thalamic pain in the face and hand. However, this operation, which the authors called "medial mesencephalotomy," affected the spino-thalamic tract also. The pains and hyperpathia were abolished and a checkup at 21 months from operation disclosed only minimal spontaneous pains.

Wycis and Spiegel (1962) performed lateral mesencephalotomy stereotactically in 16 cases of central pain. With this operation they not only destroyed the spinothalamic tract but impinged on the reticular formation of the midbrain in the region through which the second or spinoreticulothalamic pain transmission system is supposed to pass. Of the 16 cases, 14 were suffering from pains probably due to a vascular lesion, one from pain secondary to removal of a parietal cyst, and one from pain due to a hemorrhagic cystic lesion of the parietal region. In the last two cases extension of the lesion to the thalamus cannot be excluded. The immediate results were two operative deaths; 11 good results with initial disappearance or at least abatement of the pains, and three failures. In the 11 cases in which the immediate results were good the long-term results were four complete relapses in one to five months, two partial relapses in one to five months, and five lastingly good results.

They reported two other cases separately: in one case of pain from bleeding in the pons, pain was allayed for six months, whereas in the other, a patient with aneurysm of the anterior communicating artery, they obtained no improvement.

OPERATIONS ON THE THALAMUS (STEREOTACTIC THALAMOTOMY)

Hécaen *et al.* (1949) treated five cases of thalamic pain syndrome (one due to a vascular lesion; the etiology of the other four cases is unspecified) with thalamotomy. The target areas for coagulation were (a) the *center median nucleus* in one case; the patient had already been treated by injection of the sympathetic nerve and stellectomy unsuccessfully; the thalamotomy abolished the pains; the patient died four months later from bronchopneumonia; (b) *center median nucleus and adjacent part of the VPM* in three cases: immediate abolition of the pains in all three cases; one patient died a few days later without pain, the second was still well two and a half months later, and the third had a relapse after three months; (c) *center median and dorsomedian nuclei* in one case: the patient was well and pain-free five months after operation.

Baudoin and Puech (1949) treated a case of thalamic pain by injecting anesthetic into the posterior ventral nucleus but the relief was only temporary.

Spiegel *et al.* (1952) performed a thalamotomy of the VPL in three cases of thalamic pain. They obtained some relief from pain in all three cases: the result lasted for a period ranging from a few weeks to four and a half months.

Talairach *et al.* (1955) reported on 12 cases of thalamic syndrome in which the posterior ventral nucleus was destroyed stereotactically. Operative mortality was 16 percent; there was a "favorable influence" on the pains in 50 percent of the cases.

Laspiur (1956) treated two cases of thalamic syndrome from a vascular lesion by coagulating the VPL. He secured a good result

126

in one case with "practically" total disappearance of the pains. The second patient showed "spectacular" improvement of pain but a few days after the operation severe adynamia set in as a result of which the patient was discharged in precarious health and could not be followed up.

Obrador *et al.* (1957) attacked the posterior ventral nucleus in two cases of thalamic pain but obtained no immediate relief.

Hassler and Riechert (1959) treated a case of thalamic pain of vascular origin by attacking the nucleus ventralis caudalis parvicellularis and the "Medialkern." The pain was abolished but the patient died five months after operation from heart disease.

Bettag and Yoshida (1960) reported on four cases of thalamic pain due to apoplexy or to nonpenetrating head wound. Three patients were subjected to coagulation of the VPL: the immediate and long-term results were good in two cases; in the third the result was only transient. One patient was subjected to coagulation of the dorsomedian nucleus but the result was unsatisfactory. Although in the tables setting forth the data these workers reported that they had performed thalamotomy of the nucleus "ventralis caudalis" of the thalamus, in their comments on the results they stated that the best results were obtained in the cases in which they had destroyed the terminal nucleus of the spinothalamic tract and hence obviously also the nucleus ventralis caudalis parvicellularis of the classification they used.

Mark *et al.* (1960) treated a case of burning dysesthesias in all four limbs due to partial traumatic section of the cervical spinal cord. They imbedded electrodes in the VPL but they did not specify whether the pain disappeared through the mechanical lesion that this produced. Four months later they made a radiofrequency lesion, obtaining only partial relief of the pain, which returned six months later with the same characteristics as before operation.

Hassler (1960) claimed to have obtained a lasting result in four cases of thalamic pain by stereotactic coagulation of the sensory relay nuclei, the nucleus limitans, and the center median nucleus. He attributed the therapeutic success to the lesion sited in the nuclei of the diffuse projection system of the thalamus and considered these results evidence for the view that thalamic pain originates in the diffuse "trunko-thalamische" projection systems.

Bettag (1961) thought that thalamotomy at the level of the "nucleus ventralis caudalis parvicellularis" was useful in the treatment of pain.

Hankinson (1962) reported two cases of stereotactic destruction of the center median and posterior ventral nuclei for thalamic syndrome, which was successful in both cases (observation period 16–24 months).

CORTICAL OPERATIONS (PARIETAL CORTECTOMY)

Dimitri and Balado (quoted by David *et al.,* 1947) excised the ascending parietal gyrus and a large part of the superior and inferior parietal gyri on the lesion side in a case of thalamic pain without obtaining any improvement. Section of the associative fibers between the two parietal lobes at corpus callosum level was then performed but without success. A "juxta-insular" lesion affecting the corona radiata of the thalamus was found at necropsy.

Horrax (1946) reported the case (no. 3) of a 35-year-old man suffering central pain from glioma of the left hemisphere; removal of the growth did not end the pain. A parietal cortectomy was then successful, but the pains reappeared in the upper limb five months later and in the leg 14 months later. In another patient, aged 42 (no. 4), a rolandoparietal glioma removal was followed two years later by violent pain in the right hand and arm; a parietal cortectomy resulted in sedation of the pain and the good result lasted until the patient's death ten months later.

Leriche (1949) injected procaine in the postcentral gyrus of a patient suffering from thalamic pains, obtaining sedation of the pains for two months.

Stone (1950) (case cited on p. 124) reported the case of a 58-year-old woman with thalamic pains in the upper limb after vascular hemiplegia. Cervical cordotomy resulted in no improvement and even amputation of the limb at the root of the shoulder was equally unsuccessful. After this operation phantom limb pain was added to the central pain. Subpial section of the postcentral gyrus abolished the pains for the whole period of observation (14 months).

Penfield and Welch (1951) secured abolition of thalamic pains with a postcentral gyrectomy in one case but the result was not permanent and the pains gradually returned.

Lewin and Phillips (1952) reported the case of a 28-year-old patient suffering from convulsive seizures from a bullet wound in the right parietal region in whom loss of consciousness was preceded by pain in the left limbs and left side of the face. Excision of a cortical area in the parietal region had no effect on the seizures but abolished the pain.

Erickson *et al.* (1952) reported an outstandingly successful operation in a case of typical Déjerine and Roussy thalamic syndrome which arose after a stroke. The patient complained of burning pains all over the left side of the face and body. After removal of the entire postcentral gyrus the patient was pain-free for the remaining two years of his life.

Spiegel *et al.* (1954) stated that in their experience removal of the sensory cortex had no effect on thalamic hyperpathia.

White and Sweet (1955) (case quoted on p. 124) obtained a satisfactory result lasting 18 months in a case of typical thalamic syndrome which had derived no benefit from cervical cordotomy.

Rowbotham (1961) (case quoted on p. 122) performed a subpial resection of the parietal portion of the area facialis in a patient suffering from pains on one side of the head and face refractory to stellectomy and retrogasserian rhizotomy; the patient died the day after operation.

Le Beau (1954) performed frontal topectomy in three cases of thalamic syndrome. In two cases areas 9 and 10 were removed bilaterally: in one case the patient was pain-free for the four years of observation, while no improvement was obtained in the other case. The second patient was subjected to resection of the orbital gyri, which gave a little relief (two and one half years' observation). The third patient was subjected to unilateral lobotomy without success; a subsequent topectomy seems to have been successful: the patient no longer complained of pain.

White and Sweet (1955) performed complete gyrectomy of all the orbital gyri in two cases of thalamic pain.

CASE 1: A woman suffering from right orbital pains due to exenteration of the orbit for nevocarcinoma in whom trigeminal rhizotomy gave only transient relief. The rhizotomy field was then re-explored. This was followed by a vascular attack, after which the patient presented left hemiparesis and hemianalgesia followed by thalamic pains in the left trunk and limbs. Left orbital gyrectomy was performed but the relief was only transient and there was a fair degree of loss of memory and of ambition and "pep." Eight and a half months later a right orbital gyrectomy resulted in a worse memory deficit and loss of energy without relieving the pain at all; however, memory gradually recovered and the pains disappeared and the patient was still free of pain two and a half years later.

CASE 2: A woman suffering from typical thalamic syndrome after a vascular accident. Bilateral orbital gyrectomy in two stages gave no relief of pain. However, four months after operation the pains inexplicably disappeared and the patient was well.

White and Sweet (1955) performed a unilateral leucotomy on a patient with an atypical thalamic syndrome secondary to multiple embolism from rheumatic fever. The result was good: the patient sometimes felt pain but said that it no longer bothered her. The pains abated with time: five months after operation they were confined to the joints of the middle phalanges of the fingers and two years later they had disappeared completely. The patient died from peritonitis: at necropsy a right thalamic infarct and other small cerebral infarcts were found in addition, of course, to the frontal lobotomy section.

Watts and Freeman (1948) stated that they had had good results with prefrontal leucotomy in thalamic pains.

Scarff (1950) performed a left prefrontal lobotomy with good results in a patient suffering from postapoplectic thalamic pain; the good results lasted four months.

Drake and McKenzie (1953) reported that in one case in which mesencephalotomy brought on central pain a subsequent lobotomy was unsuccessful. In another patient, treated for a pain syndrome not of central origin, leucotomy gave no benefit and a subsequent mesencephalotomy brought on central pain.

Constans (1960) stated that the indications of frontal operations included the thalamic syndrome, though the results are not very brilliant.

Bonica (1954) considered that lobotomy might be useful for treating central pain from high lesions not amenable to tractotomy and that Mandl's "chemical lobotomy" may well be indicated.

Discussion

The large number of operations proposed for treating central pain is explained by the sketchiness of our knowledge of the relevant physiopathology and by the inconstant results. But however inconstant and transient the results may be, surgical treatment is still our only mean of attempting at least some temporary relief from central pain.

Our review of the literature is necessarily incomplete but a study of the material we have consulted permits us to make a few remarks that may be of interest.

It may be safely stated that some operations, such as sympathectomy, are absolutely ineffective (Turnbull, 1939; Hécaen *et al.*, 1949; White and Sweet, 1955; Rowbotham, 1961). Operations on the roots and on the peripheral nerves, performed almost exclusively for pain in the facial region (alcoholization of the gasserian ganglion or retrogasserian neurotomy), yield variable results, in the majority of cases unsatisfactory (Garcin, 1937; Frazier *et al.*, 1937; Spiegel *et al.*, 1952; White and Sweet, 1955; Rowbotham, 1961).

On the other hand, all workers are agreed that other operations have some efficacy even if only temporarily. Spinothalamic tractotomy has yielded a fair number of satisfactory results (Turnbull, 1939; White and Sweet, 1955; Frazier *et al.*, 1937; Stone, 1950; Drake and MacKenzie, 1953). According to Wycis and Spiegel (1962) stereotactic lateral mesencephalotomy can relieve thalamic pains at least temporarily (12 out of 16 cases). The same applies to stereotactic thalamotomy: of the 22 cases in the literature only two had no relief, not even to begin with (Spiegel *et al.*, 1952; Hankinson, 1962; Obrador *et al.*, 1957; Laspiur, 1956; Bettag and Yoshida, 1960; Mark *et al.*, 1960; Hassler and Riechert, 1959; Hassler, 1960; Hécaen *et al.*, 1949); unfortunately, we have not been able to consult the paper of Talairach *et al.* (1955) who reported good results in 50 percent of their cases. The immediate results of stereotactic thalamotomy operations do not seem to differ according to whether the lesion is centered on the specific relay nuclei only or whether the lesion is deliberately centered on or extends to the nuclei of the diffuse projection system. Unfortunately, in a high percentage of cases the result is only transient; furthermore, many of the cases have been followed up for too short a time for final judgment on the real efficacy of these operations.

We will now try to discuss the results of each type of operation in terms of the various theories that have been put forward to explain the pathogenesis of central pain. We feel that this is of interest since the various types of surgical operation can interrupt the pain pathways and other sensory pathways and also the polysynaptic systems. The role that these systems are thought to play in the physiopathogenesis of central pain differs according to the various theories.

Spinothalamic Tractotomy at Spinal Cord Level (Anterolateral Cordotomy) and at Bulbar Level. By means of these operations pain has been abolished in central pain syndromes due to thalamic lesions (Turnbull, 1939; Frazier *et al.*, 1937), midbrain lesions (Drake and MacKenzie, 1953), and spinal cord lesions (White and Sweet, 1955). On the other hand, apparently identical cases have derived no benefit from the operation (White and Sweet, 1955; Bohm, 1960). It is therefore impossible to draw a final conclusion regarding the usefulness or mechanism of action of this operation.

Anterolateral cordotomy interrupts (at least theoretically) the spinothalamic fibers of the paucisynaptic system that end in the thalamic relay nucleus, the spinotectal fibers, and also the long fibers of the spinoreticulothalamic system that end in the reticular systems of the brainstem and in the diffuse projection systems of the thalamus and that at spinal cord level seem to run intermixed with the fibers of the paucisynaptic system (Fig. 6). The intrinsic systems of the spinal cord—propriospinal fibers—which seem to play a major part in pain transmission are certainly interrupted, even if only by a small proportion. On the other hand, the supposed polysynaptic systems of the gelatinous substance of Rolando and the tracts of the posterior funiculi concerned with the transmission of epicritic sensibility (Fig. 9) are spared.

The therapeutic successes claimed for this operation in cases of thalamic syndrome are due, according to some workers, to the interruption of the afferent fibers coming from the periphery, which are the direct cause of the pain because they end on an "irritated" focus (thalamus) (Garcin, 1937) or one that is no longer "inhibited" and that therefore feels too keenly impulses that would normally be subliminal (Frazier *et al.*, 1937).

A continual stream of impulses from the periphery would seem to be necessary for the onset of central pain and hyperpathia, according to the irritation and liberation theories (Head and Holmes, 1911; Riddoch, 1938; Kendall, 1939) and according to those which attribute these pains to the loss of of a thalamic function subserving the elaboration of the afferent impulses (Bonhoeffer, 1938; Lhermitte, 1933; Noica and Balls, 1935; Spiegel *et al.*, 1954; Rowbotham, 1961).

Anterolateral cordotomy is justified according to these hypotheses in cases of pain from thalamic injury and in cases of hyperpathia if, as Zülch and Schmid (1953) think, the latter is due to incomplete interruption of the pain pathways but only then *if it is true that it is the impulses transmitted via the pauci-* \
synaptic systems that are responsible for central pain. However, there is no point whatever in the operation if the pain is really due to direct irritation of the sensory fibers and cells by the lesion (Déjerine and Roussy, 1906; Nicolesco, 1924). The majority of the more recent theories, which regard the polysynaptic systems, which are thought to convey pain impulses to conscious level when the paucisynaptic pathways are interrupted or functionally impaired, as the anatomic substrate of central pain (Drake and MacKenzie, 1953; Walker, 1955; Bowsher, 1960; Hassler, 1960; Noordenbos, 1959), lend no support to the operation because further damage to the paucisynaptic system would only aggravate the physiopathologic imbalance.

Open Lateral Mesencephalotomy. As far as we know, there is only one case in the literature of thalamic pain being treated by this operation. The patient died within a few hours of operation and so there are no data on which to base a discussion of the procedure.

Stereotactic Lateral Mesencephalotomy. The results obtained with this operation are good but the incidence of relapses is very high. According to Wycis and Spiegel (1962), the only workers who have used this procedure for treating central pain, only five out of 11 cases derived long-term benefit (disappearance or decrease of pain).

In this operation the spinothalamic tract (paucisynaptic pathway) should be interrupted electively. However, all the workers who have performed this operation for thalamic or other pains admit that the lesions stereotactically positioned on the lateral midbrain impinge to a greater or lesser degree on the adjacent reticular formation (Wycis and Spiegel, 1962; Roeder and Orthner, 1961; Torvik, 1961). The medial lemniscus may also be injured, as shown by the clinical observations of Spiegel and Wycis (1953) and the necropsy findings of Torvik (1959).

Section at midbrain level, in our view, differs from anterolateral cordotomy in the following ways: (1) the spinothalamic fibers, the "paucisynaptic pathway," are cut when the majority of the spinoreticular fibers (which really belong to the polysynaptic system even though they are long-tract neurons and at spinal cord level run united with them in the anterolateral funiculus) have terminated in the reticular structures of the cord, bulb, pons, and midbrain. The direct, paucisynaptic, spinothalamic contigent is cut here perhaps more completely than at cord level; fibers bound for the diffuse projection systems of the thalamus are, however, cut all the same (Fig. 6); (2) the lesion may impinge fairly extensively on the reticular formation of the brainstem; (3) the medial lemniscus runs a high risk of damage.

The remarks regarding the role of the peripheral afferent fibers and the importance of the diffuse projection systems in the causation of central pain made in connection with anterolateral cordotomy would seem to apply equally well to this operation. One may go further: for if the modern interpretations of central pain are right, then interruption of the spinothalamic tract at mesencephalic level is still less justified than cordotomy because theoretically it leaves intact the anatomic substrate that conveys central pain impulses. As we have seen, there are only five cases of therapeutic success persisting over five months. It is not improbable that the inevitable extension of the lesion to the reticular formations played an important part in these cases. Lateral mesencephalotomy is thought to act not because it interrupts the spinothalamic paucisynaptic pathways, which actually might aggravate the situation, but because it affects the polysynaptic systems. Roeder and Orthner (1961) went so far as to suggest "medial mesencephalotomy" in order to ensure more thorough interruption of the reticular formation.

Stereotactic Thalamotomy. The target of thalamotomy has varied according to the various workers. Some have attacked the sensory relay nuclei (VPL of Walker's classification, nucleus ventralis caudalis, and nucleus ventralis caudalis parvicellularis of Hassler's classification), others the nuclei of the diffuse projection system (center median nucleus, nuclei of the lamina medullaris interna, nucleus limitans according to Hassler, and so on), and yet others the two groups of nuclei together. In some cases lesions have been made in the so-called psychic integration nuclei too. We shall discuss only lesions of the first two groups of nuclei listed.

It is interesting that all workers report that good, though transient, results were obtained irrespective of the target area. This is odd if one considers the cases treated by lesions of the VPL nucleus (ventralis caudalis) and of the nucleus ventralis caudalis parvicellularis; in these cases the lesions center on the very structures damage to which is responsible, in the opinion of almost all workers, for the onset of thalamic pain: both the relay nucleus of the paucisynaptic spinothalamic system and the relay nucleus of the medial lemniscus are destroyed. A lesion of this kind is clearly a paradox in the treatment of thalamic pain or of central pain generally whatever mechanism one blames for the origin of central pain. If the thalamus analyzes, moderates, and governs pain sensation and if thalamic lesions divert pain impulses to the hypothalamus, the lesion can obviously only aggravate a central pain, especially thalamic pain; the same applies if the modern theory of the transmission of thalamic pain sensations into the

diffuse projection systems (reticulothalamic or trunko thalamische System) is true. This kind of lesion seems even more
paradoxical if we consider the experimental data, which seem to
demonstrate that the epicritic system has an inhibitory action on
the pain systems, or if the suggestion that the paucisynaptic
spinothalamic system exerts an inhibitory action on the trunko-
thalamische System is true.

Thus the only lesion that is justified by modern theories and
that even in the light of the older theories does not seem to be a
contradiction is one centering on the diffuse projection systems.
In this regard we would recall that Hassler (1960) reported good
results with lesions of the center median nucleus and its connections, of the lamina medullaris interna, and of the nucleus limitans.

How then are we to explain the good results of lesions of the
relay nuclei? It is essential to bear in mind that all the workers
who have had occasion to control postmortem the stereotactic
lesions aimed at the relay nuclei (Mark *et al.,* 1963; Maspes e
Pagni, 1965) have observed that the lesions usually go beyond
the sensory nuclei and impinge to a greater or lesser degree on
neighboring nuclei, including of necessity the nuclei of the diffuse projection system, especially the center median nucleus,
which is adjacent to the specific VPL–VPM nuclei. In all probability some of the therapeutic successes are due to the fact that
the lesions always involve, to a greater or lesser degree, the nuclei of the trunko-thalamische System.

It is easy to explain why thalamic pain is liable to relapse even
after lesions centering on and extending to the diffuse projection
systems, even assuming that they are the only lesions really
capable of yielding good results. The lesions are usually confined
to the structures on one side and are small; hence they are in a
sense partial lesions in a system whose anatomic and functional
connections are complex, extensive, and distributed over many
levels of the nervous system, from the bulb to the thalamus, a
system which cannot be put out of action completely without

causing serious impairment of all the other nervous functions.

Corticectomy. Few cases of thalamic pain have been treated in this way; however, the results seem to be good, though temporary.

Corticectomy does not seem to be justified by any of the theories so far advanced to explain central pain. The results are the more surprising if one accepts the view that cortical mechanisms are far less important than thalamic mechanisms in the conscious integration of pain (Hassler, 1960). One may well wonder whether the disappearance of the pain, temporary though it may be, is not to be ascribed to a pain "asymbolia" mechanism (Hécaen, 1957) due to the cortical lesion.

Sympathectomy. The sympathectomies reported in the literature have proved quite ineffective against thalamic and central pain. In physiopathological terms sympathectomy is like a peripheral nerve section, for there are pain fibers of the cerebrospinal pain system in the sympathetic nerve (Pellegrini and Papo, 1962). However, the physiopathological mechanism whereby the sympathetic enters into the genesis of central pain is far from clear (see Chapter 5).

Frontal Lobotomy and Leucotomy. The favorable results reported by some workers essentially concern a change in the patient's affective and psychic state. Although the data relating to these cases could be of great importance for the study of the affective component accompanying every pain syndrome, they are outside the scope of this study.

CONCLUSIONS

We will now try to summarize the most significant conclusions bearing on the pathogenesis of central pain that can, in our view, be drawn from surgical experience and briefly to compare these conclusions with those reached many years ago by the workers who first attacked this problem solely on the basis of the pathological data.

Since the time when Ajuraguerra (1937), Garcin (1937), Riddoch (1938), and Kendall (1939) attacked this problem in an organic fashion, an enormous amount has been learned about the anatomy and physiology of the systems concerned with the transmission, perception, and conscious integration of pain impulses.

During the past few years students of these questions have directed their attention more particularly to the polysynaptic or reticular systems, which, some say, extend from the posterior horns of the cord to the basal ganglia (Noordenbos, 1959; Hassler, 1960). These systems are considered to be of great importance in the transmission of sensory and pain impulses. Their role is very complex, however, for pain impulses are not only transmitted in them but undergo processes of elaboration and integration and are even brought to conscious level, or so the theory goes. In addition, and this is backed by an enormous body of experimental research (Rossi and Zanchetti, 1957), the polysynaptic systems of the more cranial portion of the brainstem play a fundamental part in the regulation of the cortical functions, for they enter into the processes of attention and all the mechanisms of the conscious integration of sensation.

We will now try to elucidate the various aspects of the problem separately.

Has surgical experience identified the systems that must be injured before a central sensory syndrome can arise?

It is clear from the study of cases of central pain caused by spontaneous lesions that, with rare exceptions, the relevant lesions involve the long pathways of pain transmission, that is the spinothalamocortical paucisynaptic pathways. Exceptional cases in which this pathway has been spared have been described in the literature. Moreover, several workers have described cases of central pain caused by lesions of Reil's band only or of the posterior funiculi only. At thalamic level there have even been cases in which the lesions are said to have spared the sensory relay nucleus (VPL–VPM) and to have been localized in the lateral posterior and lateral dorsal (LP and LD) associative nuclei.

In our opinion functional surgery for pain and extrapyramidal syndromes at spinal cord, bulb, and midbrain levels demonstrates that the *sine qua non* for central pain is a lesion of the spinothalamic system and of the quintothalamic afferences relayed through the nucleus gelatinosus of the trigeminal, that is, of the paucisynaptic system usually regarded as responsible for the transmission of pain impulses. The lesion may cause pain or in some cases only paresthesia. This pathway may be damaged at thalamocortical level also but then the lesion is not "pure" for the pathway of epicritic sensibility may be simultaneously involved. It would seem that pains and dysesthesias may also be due to lesions of the first sensory neuron at the point of entry into the neuraxis and at this level too it is impossible to say whether only the pain fibers are injured or also other sensory systems.

That an isolated lesion of the paucisynaptic pain pathway is sufficient to produce true pain is clearly demonstrated by the fact that, apart from rare and peculiar phenomena (allochiria), central sensory phenomena are always referred to territories below the level of the lesion innervated by systems of fibers of the paucisynaptic pathway, which have been damaged to a greater or lesser degree, for example, in the contralateral half of the body in pains secondary to spinothalamic tractotomy, whether performed at spinal cord or bulbar level.

In all probability damage to the paucisynaptic pathway of pain is always the necessary condition for the onset of a true central pain syndrome. We would recall that surgical experience would seem to show that lesions of the posterior funiculi alone, and hence probably of the epicritic systems only, are not enough to cause true central pain, although they can cause paresthesia.

Unfortunately, this statement is based solely on data for lesions of the posterior funiculi, that is, of the first neuron of the epicritic pathways; no cases have been reported of isolated lesions of the fibers of epicritic sensibility at the level of the brainstem, and lesions performed at thalamic level involve, as we have already pointed out, the pain fibers and the epicritic fibers simultaneously. The surgical data are thus too limited to permit the final solution of the problem as to whether pure lesions of the epicritic pathways can cause central pain.

These conclusions may seem a trifle rigid considering that there are cases in the literature that are difficult to interpret and that seem to contradict these data and in view of the fact that central pains arising after surgery have been observed almost exclusively in patients operated on for pain syndromes with techniques designed to destroy the paucisynaptic pathways.

The literature on functional surgery relating to operations that do not injure the sensory pathways yields data that may be described as "negative" but that are, we feel, of great importance.

Operations on the spinal cord, such as pyramidotomy and extrapyramidotomy, induce central pain below lesion level on the contralateral side of the body only when the section impinges on one half of the spinal cord, thereby definitely interrupting also the ascending spinothalamic pathways in the anterolateral funiculi. When the lesion is confined to other functional systems central pain does not occur. Pains with a radicular projection may, however, be produced in the course of these operations as a result of injury to the first neuron immediately after it has entered the spinal cord or to the cells of the posterior horns.

Stereotactic surgery on the thalamus similarly supplies highly significant data. Data from thousands of cases all over the world prove unequivocally that lesions which spare the sensory relay nuclei never give rise to central pain, whatever part of the thalamus is destroyed. Two observations are particularly valuable. One comes from Guiot (1964), who now coagulates even the posterior lateral nucleus (LP) for parkinsonism and who has never observed either central pain or paresthesia as a result. This experience flatly contradicts the view of Ajuraguerra (1937), who argued that lesion of a nuclear region corresponding at least in part to this nucleus was of capital importance in the generation of thalamic pain. The second vitally important observation that comes from stereotactic surgery is as follows: unless lesions of the diffuse projection system of the thalamus are associated with lesions of the sensory relay systems they cannot give rise to thalamic pain. This conclusion is based on the fact that, generally speaking, whatever portion of the thalamus is attacked stereotactically, current techniques being what they are, one inevitably impinges, to a greater or lesser degree, on the nuclei of the diffuse projection systems (lamina medullaris interna, nucleus reticularis, and so on) (Cooper *et al.,* 1963; Mark *et al.,* 1963; Macchi *et al.,* 1964; Maspes e Pagni, 1965; Pagni *et al.,* 1965). It may therefore be argued that in general lesions of the nucleus ventrolateralis performed for parkinsonism impinge to a greater or lesser extent on the diffuse projection systems and yet central pain does not occur. A similar argument could be advanced in connection with lesions of the multisynaptic systems of the spinal cord and brainstem which, as we have seen, would seem to play a part in the transmission of pain impulses: a lesion of these systems, practically inevitable in any surgical lesion of the spinal cord and brainstem, is probably not sufficient on its own to cause central pain.

One aspect of the problem on which surgery throws no direct light is central pain from cortical lesions. Although pains and hyperpathia from spontaneous parietal lesions have been reported, we have not found a single definite case of central pain from parietal gyrectomy.

In summary, surgical experience would seem to have proved that a lesion of the spinothalamocortical paucisynaptic pathway and of the quintothalamocortical afferences relayed through the nucleus gelatinosus of the trigeminal can give rise to pain, hyperpathia, and paresthesia; a lesion of the epicritic system, the spinobulbothalamocortical pathway, can probably give rise to paresthesia only and not pain; isolated lesions of the multisynaptic systems (from the spinal cord to the thalamus) cannot give rise to subjective sensory phenomena.

Granted the importance of damage to the paucisynaptic pathway (spinothalamocortical) in the genesis of central pain, is it possible to establish whether a complete interruption of this pathway is necessary?

Alongside cases of central pain in which necropsy has revealed a complete interruption of the spinothalamic tract, there are cases in which the destruction is only partial. Moreover, along with cases in which the pains are localized in completely analgesic territories, there are others in which the pains are referred to territories that are only hypoalgesic or in which the pains arise on recovery of some sensibility to heat and pain stimuli.

Is it possible to explain the different incidence of central pain from lesions at different levels of the neuraxis?

It has already been pointed out that central sensory phenomena occur more frequently in thalamic and midbrain lesions than in spinal cord and bulbar lesions. Although the surgical data cannot be statistically significant, they seem to corroborate this observation. Indeed, although there are numbers of case series of anterolateral cordotomy in which central pain was not observed, all workers who have performed operations on the thalamus and midbrain have reported central sensory phenomena in varying percentages.

It is difficult to supply an unimpeachable interpretation of these data. However, we would call attention to some anatomic and surgical evidence that may perhaps afford a basis for a physiopathological answer to this question.

Section of the anterolateral quadrant of the spinal cord interrupts a very large number of the fibers probably concerned with the transmission of pain impulses: in addition to the spinothalamic fibers proper it interrupts also the spinotectal and spinoreticular fibers which terminate in the reticular formations of the brainstem; moreover, it interrupts the impulses reaching the reticular formations of the brainstem via collaterals of the true spinothalamic long fibers that branch off from them above the level of section. Furthermore, this type of section also affects the propriospinal systems (Figs. 4, 6, and 9).

Spinothalamic tractotomy at bulbar level, which rarely gives rise to central pain, interrupts the spinothalamic, spinotectal, and spinoreticular fibers and it abolishes the transmission of impulses to the reticular formation via the collaterals that branch off from the spinothalamic fibers above the level of section.

Mesencephalotomy, which like thalamotomy carries a high incidence of central pain, spares the majority of the spinoreticular fibers and a large number of the collaterals of the spinothalamic fibers bound for the reticular substance.

Thalamotomy spares the spinoreticular, spinotectal, and all the collateral fibers of the spinothalamic long pathway.

These data show that some lesions of the so-called spinothalamic contingent interrupt to a large extent, while others leave intact, a great part of the spinoreticular afferent fibers that, at brainstem level, are bound for the system which Albe-Fessard and Fessard (1963) called the extralemniscal system. This in turn is thought to terminate in the parafascicular center median complex of the thalamus. These data may perhaps afford an anatomical basis for an explanation of the different incidence of central pain according to the level of the lesion (Fig. 6). Probably the more the surgical lesion spares the afferent fibers bound for these reticular systems of the brainstem, thereby allowing the impulses to converge on them, the greater the chances are of central sensory phenomena.

Can central sensory phenomena arise irrespective of whether the lesion affects the first, second, or third neuron of the paucisynaptic pain pathway?

We have already partially answered this question. However, at this point we would like to go into the matter more deeply, especially in regard to lesions of the first and third neurons, referring the reader to what we said earlier for lesions of the spinothalamic fibers (second neuron).

We believe it can be safely said that lesions of the first neuron can cause central pain. Indeed it is known that after Siöqvist's trigeminal tractotomy, which is designed to interrupt the central process of the cells of the gasserian ganglia after their entry into the neuraxis and before they terminate on the cells of the descending nucleus of V, postoperative paresthesias and pains may be observed in the analgesic area. Clinically these pains are indistinguishable from those due to second neuron lesions. A Siöqvist section of the descending tract of the trigeminal probably differs physiopathologically from a section of the sensory root outside the neuraxis, for the Siöqvist intramedullary section spares the fibers mediating superficial and deep sensibility and, more important, interrupts the fibers that have already given off collaterals which can reroute the pain impulses (which can no longer reach the cells of the nucleus gelatinosus, the starting point of the pain fibers bound for the quintothalamic tract) to other structures, probably reticular, which can still convey impulses to the higher centers. As Peele (1954) indicated, a very large number of trigeminal fibers on entering the pons bifurcate into an ascending and descending branch and it appears that some of these fine fibers, probably with a pain function, behave like this also and give off collaterals (Windle, 1926) (Figs. 8, 22).

Lesions of the first neuron are probably also responsible for some girdle pains from spinal cord sections performed in such a way as not to injure the sensory root outside the cord (Ebin, 1949) (see p. 91). Here again, lesion of the ascending process of the fiber, which bifurcates as soon as it enters the cord, probably prevents the pain impulses from reaching the cells of origin of the spinothalamic tract in the posterior horn but allows the impulses to escape via the descending branch or collateral branches and be transmitted to the higher centers via polysynaptic systems (Fig. 7). Thus, even at spinal cord level this section clearly has quite a different physiopathological status from that of a simple section of a peripheral root.

We shall revert to the possibility of diversion of impulses onto the reticular systems when we deal with the theories that account for the origin of central pain.

In regard to the third neuron of the paucisynaptic pathway, or the thalamoparietal neuron, we feel we can safely say that lesion of this can also give rise to central pain. Indeed, whereas in thalamic lesions it is impossible to say whether the onset of pain is due to lesion of the thalamic neuron or of the secondary fiber afferent to it, we feel it is impossible to doubt the importance of lesion of the thalamoparietal neuron in cortical lesions, whether one attributes the pain to lesion of the cortical sensory area or whether, as some workers believe, the pain is due to phenomena of retrograde degeneration of the thalamic neurons. The fact that after surgical operations on the parietal cortex no central pains are observed may be explained by the fact that the cortical pain projection area is probably rather circumscribed and confined to a small area of the upper lip of the sylvian fissure (Hassler, 1960; Biemond, 1956) and so is spared by these operations which are designed to remove a circumscribed area of the ascending parietal gyrus. The higher incidence of central pain from spontaneous parietal lesions is probably due to the fact that pathologic lesions may involve the supposed cortical pain area.

Let us now sum up the points that we feel are definitely established: (a) for central pain to arise, a lesion of the cells or long fibers of the paucisynaptic pain system, the spinothalamocortical fibers proper (Fig. 3a), seems to be necessary; (b) inside the neuraxis it does not seem to matter whether the first, second, or third neuron is affected; (c) central pain may occur as a result of partial or total lesion of the spinothalamic tract; (d) isolated lesions of the spinoreticulothalamic polysynaptic system (Figs. 3b and c) do not seem to be sufficient to give rise to true central pain; and (e) pure lesions of the pathways of epicritic sensibility—spinobulbothalamocortical or so-called lemnyscal system—at least as regards the first neuron, do not seem to give rise to central pain but only to paresthesias.

Assuming that the anatomic premises we have outlined are valid, which of the theories put forward to explain the occurrence of central pain are acceptable and which are not?

If a lesion, partial or total, of the afferent paucisynaptic pain system at any level of the neuraxis is sufficient to induce central pain, certain theories would seem to break down.

The theory of Head and Holmes (1911), which attributes the pains to hyperirritability of the thalamic nuclei or of the subthalamic nuclei (Foerster, 1927) released from a cortical control, is no longer tenable because a lesion of the corticofugal pathways does not seem to be necessary.

The theories which attribute to the epicritic system a damping action on the pain transmission system (Riddoch and Critchley, 1937; Frazier *et al.,* 1937; Riddoch, 1938) and which regard central sensory phenomena as the consequence of altered functional relations between the two systems would seem to be equally groundless. As we have already pointed out, cases of "pure" surgical lesions of the epicritic system are few and confined to the first neuron, but nevertheless, none of the workers who have performed them has ever observed true central pain. This conclusion may appear a little arbitrary when there is electrophysiological evidence to support the above theories (Poggio and Mountcastle, 1960); but there are too many examples of central pain from surgical lesions that definitely spare the lemniscal pathway, such as anterolateral cordotomy and bulbar spinothalamic tractotomy, for this mechanism to be regarded as having a constantly pre-eminent role.

Theories according to which the thalamus exerts a "restraining," "damping," or "filter" action on normal pain sensations (Lhermitte, 1933; Noica and Balls, 1935) might account for pains from thalamic but not from subthalamic lesions. These theories may have some real foundation, for sensory stimuli do undergo some elaboration at thalamic level before reaching the cortex and, according to some workers, pain stimuli may actually be consciously integrated there.

A group of theories that would seem to be unassailable are those based on irritation: no one can rule out the possibility that fibers and cells at lesion level undergo an irritative process and that this is one of the fundamental factors in the genesis of central pain.

With regard to theories based on the sympathetic system, perhaps the autonomic system plays a part in the genesis of central pain, but the mechanisms at work are far from clear and most workers consider that the sympathetic system plays a secondary part. It would seem to be definite that central pain can occur without clinical evidence of autonomic involvement.

A group of theories deserving rather fuller discussion are those which attribute central pain to the transmission of pain stimuli along the polysynaptic slow systems of the spinal cord, brainstem, and thalamus (Drake and MacKenzie, 1953; Walker, 1955; Bowsher, 1960), which, according to some workers (Kendall, 1939; Noordenbos, 1959; Hassler, 1960), are kept under the damping or inhibitory influence of the paucisynaptic systems. Whether or not that is so, according to these theories central pain occurs because stimuli are conveyed along a system whose physiological function is to transmit pain sensations of an aching character poorly localized in time and place. After lesions of the paucisynaptic system, the polysynaptic slow system is thought to come to the fore either because it is released from the damping action of the injured system or simply because, the other system being injured, it functions alone.

These theories accord perfectly with the anatomic data that we have gathered from surgical experience of central pain and they may account for the different incidence of central pain according to the site of the lesions. And if, as Noordenbos (1959) believed, the paucisynaptic system has an inhibitory action on the polysynaptic system, they provide an explanation of all, even the oddest, aspects of central sensory phenomena.

With regard to the problem of the different incidence of central pain according to the level of the lesion, Fig. 6 sums up what we have already said. The higher the level of the lesion, the greater the number of afferent impulses that may be diverted to the diffuse projection formations and hence the greater the activation of the trunko-thalamische System. This is probably why the incidence of central pain is greatest for thalamomesencephalic lesions.

Another problem that these theories may help to solve is the importance of sensory afferent impulses in the genesis of central pain. Clearly, only theories based on irritation can account for this without incriminating the peripheral afferent fibers. All the other theories, even if the authors do not explicitly mention it, of necessity presuppose an incessant bombardment of impulses from the periphery. While for some workers these impulses must be pain impulses, for others they are not necessarily so, some considering that they may actually be any afferent sensory impulse. It has rightly been pointed out, however, that if stimuli from the periphery are necessary for the occurrence of central pain, it is odd, to say the least, that these pains should be referred to totally or globally anesthetic areas. As early as 1953 Zülch and Schmid thought that some areas were not actually anesthetic and that there were still some sensory endings functioning though able to respond only to massive and diffuse stimulation.

Even from areas that are clinically anesthetic for all modalities—as after a thalamic lesion, for instance—normal stimuli still reach the posterior horns of the spinal cord incessantly. These stimuli do not reach conscious level because the fast point-by-point projection pathways, that is paucisynaptic pathways, have been interrupted but they are still conveyed by collaterals of the fibers (first and second neurons) and by spinoreticular fibers to the polysynaptic systems of the spinal cord and brainstem. Given the nature of the multisynaptic system, these impulses, which lose their spatial localization and sequence in time (Nathan, 1955), are responsible for the abnormal sensations of central sensory syndromes.

This is how the role of the peripheral afferent fibers is explained. Certain characteristics of central pains can also be explained by these theories. Assuming that the paucisynaptic system does exert a damping action on the polysynaptic systems (as Noordenbos, for example, believes), it is easy to see why central pains can be precipitated by non-pain and by sensory stimuli, by stimuli coming from regions belonging to dermatomes distant from those to which the pains are referred. It is well known that there is a multisensory convergence (Albe-Fessard and Fessard, 1963) on the cells of certain nuclei of the polysynaptic systems of the brainstem (for example, the giant cell nucleus of the brainstem and the center median nucleus of the thalamus) and if the conception of the spinoreticulothalamic polysynaptic system is correct, it is obvious that impulses conveyed along that system from lower levels will converge on every segment of the system right from the lowest levels of the cord. A "local disinhibition" (Noordenbos, 1959) of the polysynaptic system, due to reduction of the number of impulses normally conveyed to a given point of this system by the A fibers of the peripheral nerve and by fibers of the spinothalamic system and its collaterals, induces hypersensitivity of this neuron pool and so any other stimulus reaching this hyperesthetic neuron pool causes a pain which is referred to the territory innervated by the damaged peripheral nerve or to a territory innervated by the fibers of the interrupted paucisynaptic system, and so on.

This is the mechanism that Noordenbos (1959) invoked to account for central pain, which may thus be due to impulses generated outside the segment of the body to which the pain is referred. They are the slow impulses running upwards in the multisynaptic system, which have lost their localizing and functional significance because of the characteristics of the system transmitting them "owing to the many ramifications of the system" (Noordenbos, 1959) and which on reaching a disinhibited or partially disinhibited "neuron pool" induce pain.

In conclusion, although there is no final proof as to which mechanisms are responsible for central pain, we feel that these modern theories emphasizing the importance of the polysynaptic systems account for many of the clinical features of these pains and that they supply a fairly sound anatomicophysiological basis for a plan of research designed to elucidate these problems. We consider that an exhaustive clinical and histopathological study of all cases subjected to functional surgery, and not only of the cases in which central pain arose, might supply the final answer to a number of questions.

As indicated in the chapter on symptomatology, patients suffering from central pain complain of several kinds of disagreeable sensations, both spontaneous and precipitated by peripheral stimuli. Is the same physiopathological mechanism at work both in spontaneous and in induced phenomena?

As far as we know, the only workers who maintain that spontaneous and induced pains cannot be explained by the same physiopathological mechanism are Sokolianski and Kulkova

(1938). Other workers have not bothered to distinguish between the two. Furthermore, as we have already mentioned, the nomenclature is used differently by different workers and this gives rise to great confusion.

It is important to remember that spontaneous and induced pains have similar characteristics and that the two are often associated in the same patient and even coexist or succeed one another in a given district of the body.

We believe it possible that the two phenomena have a common physiopathological mechanism. If the peripheral afferent stimuli are necessary to keep in being pains due to lesion of the central nervous system, this hypothesis seems more than likely. If it is correct, then what is commonly called spontaneous pain is not really so, since it is kept up by physiologic (interoceptive and exteroceptive) peripheral stimuli that in the healthy individual do not cause pain or do not surface to conscious level. In some patients these stimuli cause "spontaneous" pain, while in others they are not strong enough to do so and only new stimuli—more intense, prolonged and repeated or diffuse—can produce pains that are then called "induced." But the anatomicophysiological substrate is the same in both cases.

To illustrate this point let us take the case of a patient with cancer pain subjected to stereotactic thalamotomy of the VPL nucleus; the pains for which he has been operated on disappear but central pains of an apparently spontaneous type come on. Clearly, the peripheral lesion remains unchanged and with it the flow of pain impulses, but these are no longer experienced consciously with the usual characteristics of intensity, localization and duration because the specific paucisynaptic pathway has been interrupted; they still reach the higher centers via the spinoreticulothalamic polysynaptic system and are felt by the consciousness as having the characteristics of central pains, apparently "spontaneous" but in reality induced.

In apparent contrast to this situation there is the case of a healthy individual in whom a vascular lesion of the thalamus causes a thalamic syndrome with only pains of the "induced" type, that is, only intense and prolonged peripheral stimulation induces pain. At a physiopathological level there does not seem to us to be any difference between these two cases: the pain stimuli induced by the tumoral invasion of the nervous pathways in the first patient have exactly the same status as the intense and massive pain stimuli induced by the examiner in the second patient, the only difference being the duration of stimulation. As we have already mentioned, in some patients habitual stimuli, such as the contact with clothing, and so on, are sufficient to bring on the pains, which are only apparently spontaneous.

At this point one may well ask why stimuli that are normally not painful induce central pains in some patients and in others not. This probably depends on individual factors and we shall refer to this problem later on.

Is the physiopathological mechanism responsible for the onset of central pain always the same irrespective of the level of the neuraxis at which fibers of the paucisynaptic pain system are injured?

We have to some extent already answered this question, but we will now briefly summarize the salient features of the problems. As early as 1937 Garcin had raised the question but he did not go into it.

It seems that central pain can arise as a result of lesions of the first, second, or third neurons of the paucisynaptic pathway within the neuraxis. Whatever the lesion, there is always the possibility that pain impulses arrested in their progress through the paucisynaptic system will be diverted on to the ascending multisynaptic systems of the spinal cord, brainstem, and thalamus (Figs. 6, 7). In lesions of the first neuron the pain impulses can be switched onto the polysynaptic systems via the collaterals and main branches of the fibers of the sensory root that may have been spared by the injury. In lesions of the second and third neurons, that is, from the posterior horns of the cord to the thalamus,

153

the higher the level of the lesion, the greater the chances of pain impulses being diverted by collaterals or by fibers bound for the reticular formation to the multisynaptic formations.

In our opinion this possibility of diverting pain impulses onto the multisynaptic formations is the common denominator of all central pain. The different incidence of pains according to the level of the lesion may, as we have already said, be due to the fact that with certain lesions the number of fibers afferent to the poly-synaptic systems that are spared and hence able to convey pain impulses to these systems is small (lesions of the first and of the second neurons at spinal cord level), whereas with others (mes-encephalotomy and lesions of the relay nucleus of the thalamus) the convergence of the impulses on the multisynaptic systems is completely preserved (Figs. 6, 7): in the former case the inci-dence of central pain is a rare occurrence, in the latter it is a fre-quent one.

In short, we think that the anatomicophysiological substrate necessary for the onset of central pain is always the same what-ever the site of the lesion responsible. This fact might explain why the clinical features of central pain may be identical irre-spective of lesion level (first, second, or third neurons). Apart from the workers who have studied the problem of central pain from thalamic lesions only, all those who have studied the physiopathological mechanism of central pain have regarded it as the same for any level, though they have not sought an explanation.

Problems that remain unsolved are (1) given the same lesion, why do central pains arise only in some patients and not in all? (2) why is there such variability in time of onset?

There are many sides to these problems: probably histo-pathologic factors (mode of evolution of the healing reactions, individual tissue reactions) and functional factors that are dif-ficult to assess (diaschisis, individual predisposition, different synaptic permeability of certain neuronal systems, pre-existence of pain syndromes) come into play.

Garcin (1937) regarded irritative phenomena as fundamental in the genesis of central pains. He considered that the different type of anatomicopathological lesion and the different type of tissue reaction from individual to individual were factors of prime importance. Actually these factors may be important in accounting for the different time of onset and whether or not they later disappear. The tissue readjustments that take place in time during the evolution of a scar are probably of great importance: during a repair process some fibers put out of action by the acute attack may recover their activity or, with the evolution and extension of a glial scar, other fibers functioning until then may be permanently impaired.

The difference in time of onset of the pains can very probably be explained partly by functional mechanisms, for phenomena of diaschisis, which may totally block function within one or several systems, may vary in duration from subject to subject. Moreover, if it is true that the onset of central pain necessarily implies the transmission of impulses through the polysynaptic systems, systems which in normal conditions probably have a minor or vicarious function in pain transmission, it is easy to understand that the coming into operation of this secondary system may require longer in some people than in others. In other words, the different degree of synaptic permeability of this system, which usually has an ancillary function, might account for the difference in time of onset of the pains. This may be the determining factor in what is known as individual predisposition.

How are central pain phenomena to be treated?
It is well known that medical therapy has no effect upon these pains; therefore, great hopes were placed on surgical methods. Yet, as the literature shows, there is no surgical method that can guarantee permanent or even temporary relief. None of the

155

operations so far tried has yielded relief in more than a varying percentage of cases, and then as a rule only temporarily or partially; in a large number of cases the result has been total failure.

In the great majority of cases the purpose of these operations has been to interrupt the paucisynaptic pain pathways (anterolateral cordotomy, lateral mesencephalotomy, thalamotomy of the VPL and VPM); less frequently the aim has been to interrupt also the polysynaptic systems either in isolation (thalamotomy of the center median nucleus, medial mesencephalotomy) or in association with the paucisynaptic pathways (thalamotomy of the center median nucleus and of the VPM and VPL).

After what has been said about the probable pathogenesis of central pain, especially in the light of the most up-to-date concepts of the function of the multisynaptic systems, it is clear that lesions of the paucisynaptic are probably a contradiction in terms, since it is a lesion of this system that is responsible for central pain. Certain types of operation would be justified solely in the case in which the central pains were to be attributed to "partial" lesions of the pain pathways, as Zülch and Schmid (1953) maintained. In this case the complete interruption of these pathways should systematically abolish hyperpathic pain, but surgical experience does not bear out this hypothesis.

It is more likely that central pain has its anatomicophysiological substrate in the polysynaptic systems. Hence, therapeutic lesions should probably aim at interrupting the transmission of pain stimuli in these systems. This is the principle underlying the "medial mesencephalotomy" proposed by Roeder and Orthner (1961). But, in view of the anatomicofunctional situation of these systems and their extent, it is virtually impossible to effect lesions that are extensive enough and such as to ensure sufficient stoppage of the transmission of pain stimuli without causing severe functional disorders (disturbances of alertness, consciousness, and so on). The lesions that a surgeon can effect in these systems without bringing on unpleasant side-effects can only be partial lesions likely to bring vicarious mechanisms into play. For technical reasons (greater ease of access and less risk of impinging on vital neighboring structures), it is easier to attempt a lesion of these polysynaptic systems at the level of the center median nucleus of the thalamus. Unfortunately, not even stereotactic lesions at this level have always given a satisfactory result, probably because of the smallness of the lesion. No bilateral lesions have ever been effected in the center median nucleus. Because it is impossible to effect massive lesions of these systems in a single operation, it is natural to speculate whether such lesions, including bilateral lesions and lesions extending to other nuclei of the diffuse projection system, could not be effected in stages.

Peripheral radicotomy needs to be discussed separately. This would be the only operation indicated were central pain due to impulses from the periphery diverted and transmitted via the polysynaptic systems. Actually, the operation has been performed only for central pains localized in the face. The results of retrogasserian rhizotomy have been excellent in some cases.

There is no surgical experience of radicotomy for central pains referred to the limbs or trunk. It would be interesting if there were because this operation should be completely effective, if central pain were due simply to the fact that once the paucisynaptic spinothalamic system is put out of action there remains in operation only the polysynaptic system, which thus comes to the fore and brings to conscious level only abnormal, dull, aching sensations, *due to impulses coming from the dermatomes to which the pain is referred.* But if the cause of the pain lies in the abolition of the inhibitory action exerted on the polysynaptic slow system at any level of the nervous system by the fast fibers not only of the spinothalamic system but also of the peripheral nerve (Noordenbos, 1959), radicotomy, by abolishing altogether the afferent portions of the fast A fibers, would only aggravate the situation. Indeed, after radicotomy the multisynaptic system is still always "activated" by impulses ascending through the polysynaptic system itself or even coming from contralateral segments of the body. Hence, impulses continue to bombard the area of the polysynaptic system "disinhibited" by lesions of the fast pathways and so hyperesthetic; central pain would continue, therefore, despite radicotomy.

In cerebrospinal operations for pain syndromes is it possible to prevent the onset of central pain?

If the theoretical premises that we have outlined and discussed are valid, one is driven to the conclusion that it is virtually impossible with the classic operations of cerebrospinal surgery to rule out the risk of central pain. Hence spinal cord, bulbar, and mesencephalic tractotomy and stereotactic lesions aimed at the VPM and VPL, all operations designed to interrupt the paucisynaptic pain pathway, should theoretically be discontinued. In the present state of our knowledge it is impossible to be sure that central pain will not arise after one of these operations and the surgeon cannot conceal this risk from the patient, a risk which, as we have seen, varies percentage-wise with the type of operation and, if it materializes, sometimes brings pains that are worse than the ones for which the patient was operated on.

These considerations are of the utmost importance if the patients contemplating surgery for a pain syndrome have a long life expectancy, for, as we have seen, central pain can arise quite some time after operation. The problem of treating intractable pain remains an almost daily problem for the neurosurgeon. If certain cerebrospinal operations are still justifiable today in patients with cancer and a short life expectancy, it is debatable whether one of these operations should be performed in patients suffering from pain syndromes of other etiology. Probably stereotactic operations centering on the diffuse projection systems and chemical radicotomy, now being tried out experimentally, are the two avenues open to the treatment of pain syndromes.

APPENDIX

The authors are indebted to Dr. Erwin Wildi of the Institut de Pathologie, Geneva, for the necropsic and histologic study of cases 1 and 2.

CASE 1

De M.T., a 50-year-old man. Pancoast's syndrome from tumor of apex of right lung. One-year history of pains in right upper limb, upper right chest, and right side of neck. Hyperesthesia of upper half of right chest and of right upper limb. Cobalt therapy gave poor results.

Operation. Repérage of center median (CM) nucleus and nucleus ventralis posterior lateralis (VPL) on left side with Talairach's stereotactic apparatus in general anesthesia. Insertion of one 1-mc. granule of ^{90}Y in each of the target structures.

Postoperative course. Gradual disappearance of pains in 3 days. On third day, hypesthesia to light touch, heat, and pain throughout the right side of the body including the face; total loss of position sense, astereognosis, partial loss of vibration sense. Patient was discharged on the eighth day completely free of pain. Six weeks after operation patient began to suffer from a pain symptom-complex different in site and nature from the one for which he had been operated on. The pain, which spread to the right side of the face and the whole of the right chest, later spread to the right upper limb. This new pain, completely different from the previous one, was a typical thalamic pain. The symptom-complex lasted until the patient's death five months after operation as the result of a bronchopneumonia episode due to an esophagotracheal fistula.

Necropsy. In the inferior posterior part of the pulvinar there was a necrosis, 1.5 cm long at the greatest diameter, lying obliquely

159

in front of the posterior commissure. It was a yellowish-gray necrosis very well demarcated by a small ochre-colored layer; the center of the necrosis was also pigmented. The lesion had almost totally destroyed the posterior portion of the thalamus. It affected the relay sensory nuclei: the VPL nucleus was totally destroyed and only a very small part of the VPM was spared. The center median nucleus (CM) was extensively destroyed. The lesion impinged on the mid-line nuclei, the lamina medullaris interna, grazed the internal capsule, impinged extensively on the lateral posterior (LP) nucleus, and destroyed a small part of the dorsomedian nucleus (DM). (For histologic findings see Maspes e Pagni, 1965, case no. 12.) (Fig. 25.)

FIG. 25. Case 1. Anatomic specimen showing the very large lesion stereotactically placed in the posterior half of the left thalamus, which gave rise to central pain. (See text for further information.) *Source:* Maspes and Pagni (1965).

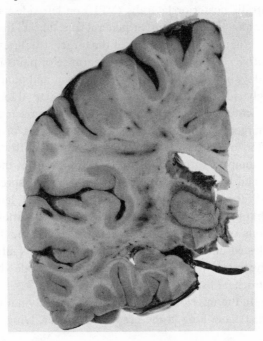

CASE 2

T.A., a 58-year-old man. Sarcoma of the left parotid region. Eleven-month history of swelling behind the left mandible. Ten-month history of continuous pain in the region behind the left ear radiating to the back of the neck, cervical region, and left jaw. Very high doses of cobalt therapy gave no relief. Tongue and jaw movements restricted for some months; difficulty in swallowing. No deficit of sensibility. Obliged to use analgesics, but they gave no relief whatever.

Operation. An operation in local anesthesia was attempted but patient was uncooperative. Operation had to be interrupted because of cardiocirculatory failure. Twelve days later repérage of nucleus ventralis posterior lateralis (VPL), nucleus ventralis posterior medialis (VPM), and the center median nucleus on the right side with Talairach's stereotactic apparatus, in general anesthesia. The target structures were coagulated. The VPL and VPM nuclei were coagulated because the pain affected not only the face but in the most violent bouts the cervical region also.

Postoperative course. Total and immediate disappearance of pain. Postoperative sensibility tests showed hypesthesia to light touch, heat, and pain in the left side of the body, including the face, deep sensibility and stereognosis totally abolished on the left side of the body. Left corneal reflex diminished. On the 13th day the sense deficit on the left side of the body was unchanged and the cervicofacial pains were absent. It was noted, however, for the first time, that stimuli of all kinds applied to the left side gave rise to a "disagreeable" sensation, vague in character, that spread out from the point of stimulation. In the next few days a spontaneous "thalamic" pain set in. The patient complained of a continuous and tiresome burning sensation all over the left side of the body, which persisted until his death on the 56th day as a result of a bout of bronchopneumonia ab ingestis due to the difficulty of swallowing.

Necropsy. The lesion of the right thalamus appeared on a cut passing 2 mm in front of the point at which the gray commissure should be found (absent in this case); hence the whole of the anterior half of the thalamus was intact. Less than 1 cm behind there were three confluent necroses: on the horizontal plane the greatest diameter of the three lesions was 3 cm and the width 1 cm. Laterally the lesion impinged slightly on the posterior portion of the internal capsule. The lateral geniculate body was separated from the outermost lesion by 3 mm of white substance, apparently intact. Medially the lesion arrived within 2 mm of the ependyma and within 4 mm of the visible part of the posterior white commissure. In the next section the three lesions are seen to extend as far as the pulvinar where the two outermost lesions still run together, while the most medial is close to the superior colliculus.

The lesions affected the following structures:

(a) nuclei VPL and VPM: the VPM nucleus was nearly totally destroyed; only a part of the VPL nucleus was destroyed;

(b) the CM nucleus, which was nearly completely destroyed;

(c) the medial lemniscus;

(d) the lamina medullaris interna, the nucleus reticularis, the LP nucleus, the nuclei medialis and lateralis pulvinaris, the medialis dorsalis, the nucleus ventralis lateralis, which were partially destroyed.

The lesion impinged also on a small part of the posterior limb of internal capsulae (Fig. 26).

(For histologic findings see Maspes e Pagni 1965, case no. 17)

CASE 3

B.D., a 54-year-old woman. Painful trigeminal anesthesia after rhizotomy. Subjected to Frazier's retrogasserian neurotomy in November 1959 for trigeminal neuralgia affecting branches I and II on the left. This operation left the patient with left facial hypesthesia to all modalities. She kept well for three months and then continuous deep pains appeared in the left side of the palate irradiating to the left zygomatic and supraorbital regions, with paroxysmal exacerbations. In May 1960 the patient was subjected to Dandy's posterior neurotomy, which left her with total anesthesia on the left side of the face without reducing the pain. For the next three years the pain continued unabated.

Operation. Using Talairach's stereotactic technique in local anesthesia the VPM and CM nuclei on the right side were coagulated after stimulation.

Postoperative course. Immediate and total abolition of the pain in the left side of the face; onset of anesthesia for deep sensibility throughout the left side of the body with severe hypesthesia to light touch, heat and pain. (The face was already anesthetic to all modalities before operation.) On the sixth day a spontaneous pain syndrome came on, with thalamic hyperpathia on the left side of the body but not in the face; these symptoms gradually abated and ceased altogether spontaneously on the 21st day.

CASE 4

T.R., a 37-year-old man. An injury to the left brachial plexus left the patient with monoplegia and causalgia of the left upper

FIG. 26. Case 2. Anatomic specimen showing the lesions stereotactically placed in the right thalamus, which gave rise to central pain. (See text for further information.) *Source:* Maspes and Pagni (1965).

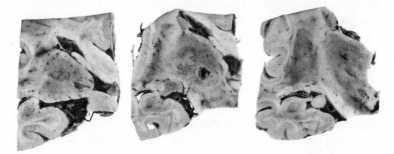

limb. On testing for cutaneous resistance there were signs of total sympathetic denervation in the left upper limb. Severe hypesthesia to all modalities in C5, C6, and C7 on left with patches of anesthesia.

Operation. Using Talairach's technique in local anesthesia, the CM, VPL, and Reil's band immediately below thalamic level were coagulated on the right side after stimulation.

Postoperative course. In the first few postoperative days the patient was slightly drowsy but the spontaneous pains were completely abolished. There was severe hypesthesia to light touch, heat, pain, and deep sensibility all over the left side of the body. There was total paralysis of left upper limb (already present before operation) and mild paresis of the left lower limb; but the functional deficit was aggravated considerably by the concomitant disturbance of deep sensibility. By the eighth day the pains in the upper limb had totally disappeared but a typical thalamic hyperpathia appeared in the left side of face and chest and the left leg. There was then a slow but steady relapse of the pains that had brought the patient to operation and the thalamic hyperpathia persisted, though apparently to a somewhat lesser degree. A neurological checkup 15 months after operation showed very severe hemihypesthesia on the left, face included, to all modalities; typical thalamic hyperpathia in the left side of the face and chest and in the left leg with spontaneous pains; pains reappeared in the left arm and were almost as severe as before operation, though it is impossible to say whether they constituted a relapse or were part of the central pain syndrome. The stimuli that precipitated hyperpathic phenomena in the other bodily districts did not do so in the upper limb.

CASE 5

F.V., a 63-year-old woman. Painful trigeminal anesthesia after Frazier's rhizotomy. Patient had been suffering from right facial neuralgia for seven years. She was subjected to Frazier's retrogasserian neurotomy in September 1963: immediate abolition of the pains and onset of total anesthesia in branches I and II and of hypesthesia to all modalities in III. About 15 days after operation a continuous painful burning sensation came on in the right side of the face. According to the patient the pains were unbearable and analgesics afforded no relief.

Operation. Using Talairach's technique in local anesthesia, coagulation of the left center median (CM) nucleus after stimulation, which gave rise to sensory phenomena on the left side of the body, mainly in the hand but never in the face.

Postoperative course. Immediate abolition of pains in the right side of the face. The patient was slightly disoriented and lightheaded. Clinical examination disclosed total anesthesia to all modalities in the right hand and forearm; hypesthesia to all modalities in the right arm and lower limb; sensibility of trunk unaffected; sensory responses of the right side of the face unchanged; pronounced ataxic syndrome of the right upper limb. Patient quickly regained her mental balance. By the eighth postoperative day she began to have deep pains affecting practically all the right half of the body but worse in the upper limb. During the next three weeks the pains were referred only to the upper limb, where the sensory deficit was worst, and to the right side of the chest. The pains were deep, gnawing, poorly localized, and were accentuated by light pricking stimuli. After an additional two months the patient complained again of burning pains in the right side of the face.

CASE 6

C.M., a 53-year-old man. Carcinoma of the left parotid region. Intractable pains in the left side of the face and head. About a year before admission pains commenced in the left side of the jaw; later a large swelling arose behind the left jaw, with dysphagia. Roentgentherapy was given. The clinical findings on admission were: the large swelling behind the jaw was ulcerated (roentgen lesion) and surrounded by radiodermatitis; left trismus; peripheral paralysis of VII on left; hypesthesia extending to virtually the whole of the left trigeminal territory; very severe left craniofacial pains which were refractory to analgesics. The patient was a confirmed alcoholic.

Operation. Using Talairach's technique in local anesthesia repérage and coagulation of the right center median (CM) nucleus after stimulation, which gave rise to sensory responses in the left hand. The coordinates were calculated for the right VPM and an electrode-bearing screw was set over that nucleus. The coordinates for the left CM were calculated and an electrode-bearing screw was set there. A depth electrode was inserted through the inner bore of the screw, the tip of the electrode reaching the left CM nucleus.

Postoperative course. Immediate abolition of pain. Clinical examination disclosed no sensory deficits (apart from the craniofacial hypesthesia described). On the fifth day the patient became increasingly drowsy. The depth electrode on the left CM target was extracted and the drowsiness disappeared completely within a few hours. On the 11th day the patient complained anew of pains at the level of the internal auditory canal, which increased and extended as the days went by. It was decided to effect another coagulation, this time of the right VPM. Stimulation of the target area produced sensory phenomena on the left side of the body but not on the face. Using the indwelling electrode-bearing screw referred to previously, this target area was coagulated. Cessation of the spontaneous pain and immediate onset of painful stabbing sensations all over the left side of the body but not the face, with awkwardness in the movements of the limbs. Hypesthesia all over the left side of the body (the face was already hypesthetic before operation). During the next few days the craniofacial pains were still absent, but the mild thalamic dysesthesias remained. Follow-up one month after the second coagulation showed no change.

CASE 7

L.A., 63-year-old woman. Facial paraspasm of over five years' duration.

Operation. Using Talairach's stereotactic apparatus in local anesthesia coagulation of the right CM nucleus after stimulation, which evoked sensory responses in the upper limb and in the left side of the face.

Postoperative course. The facial paraspasm disappeared immediately and was absent for 5 days, after which there was total relapse. On the tenth day the patient complained of spontaneous dysesthesias on left side of the face (cold, feeling of swollenness, she felt as if her skin were made of cardboard) and in the left hand; teeth-cleaning and nail-filing precipitated mild pains in these regions. Clinical examination disclosed hypesthesia to light touch, heat, pain, and to deep stimuli in the third and fourth fingers of the left hand; stimuli were felt on the left side of the face but with a "perverted" character. Patient was not unduly bothered by these sensory phenomena and was able to carry on her normal way of life for the seven months during which she was followed up.

CASE 8

N.D., a 40-year-old man. Injury to the left brachial plexus. Causalgia on the ulnar side of the volar aspect of the forearm, the palm of the hand and the volar aspect of the fourth and fifth fingers of the left hand. Anesthesia from C4 to T2 on the left. Surgical exploration of the brachial plexus showed that it was completely torn, with an irreparable lesion of the roots of the plexus. Phenol blockade of the epidural space at C5–C6 was unsuccessful.

Operation. Repérage of the right subcortical thalamoparietal sensory projections by Talairach's technique. Three granules of radioactive yttrium laid at the points of the projection where stimulation gave rise to sensory phenomena in the left upper limb.

Postoperative course. Immediate cessation of the pains; onset of global hypesthesia to all modalities throughout the left side of the body, including the face, and hypesthesia of the left lower limb with hypotonia. The patient was free of pain on discharge on the 28th day. Three months after operation he began to suffer from a new type of spontaneous pain all over the left upper limb but mainly in the shoulder, neck and chest on the left side. The pains, which the patient described as "excruciating," affected regions which were not affected by the original pains. These symptoms were continuing 16 months after operation: the pains for which patient had been operated on had disappeared but it was not clear whether these new pains affected the ulnar volar aspect of the forearm and fingers as well.

BIBLIOGRAPHY

Adams, R. D., and D. Munro (1944). "Surgical Division of the Spinothalamic Tract in the Medulla," *Surg. Gynec. Obstet.*, 78: 591–
599.

Ajuraguerra de, J. (1937). *La douleur dans les affections du système
nerveux central* (Paris: Doin).

———— and H. Hécaen (1954). "Syndrome thalamique," in *Encyclo-
pédie médico-chirurgical Française Neurologie*, I, 17037 F. 10.
(Paris: Masson).

Alajouanine, Th., and R. Thurel (1944); quoted by M. David, *et al.*
(1947).

———— and A. Brunelli (1935). "Les douleurs alternés dans les lé-
sions bulbo-protubérantielles. Contribution à l'étude de la physiopathologie des douleurs centrales," *Rev. neurol.*, 63:828–837.

Albe-Fessard, D., and A. Fessard (1963). "Thalamic Integrations and
Their Consequences at the Telencephalic Level," in *Brain Mech-
anisms*, ed. G. Moruzzi, A. Fessard, and H. H. Jasper (Amsterdam:
Elsevier Publ. Co.), pp. 115–154.

Amici, R. (1955). "Contributo clinico allo studio dei blastomi dei
nuclei ottico-striati. 20 osservazioni personali," *Sist. nerv.*, 7:260–
300.

Antonucci, O. (1938). "Chordotomia posterior medialis (dei cordoni
di Goll) nelle paraplegie spastiche (tipo Little)," *Policlinico, Sez.
prat.*, 39:1761–1768.

Armour, (1927); quoted by P. Wertheimer and J. Lecuire (1953).

Babtchine, I. S. (1936). "Les résultats immédiats et lointains de la
cordotomie," *J. Chir.* (Paris), 47:26–39.

Bailey, R. A., P. Glees, and D. R. Oppenheimer (1954). "Midbrain
Tractotomy: A Surgical and Clinical Report with Observations on
Ascending and Descending Tract Degeneration," *Mschr. Psychiat.
Neurol.*, 127:316–335.

Baudoin, A., and J. Lhermitte (1932), quoted by Riddoch, 1938.

Baudoin, A., and P. Puech (1949). "Premiers essais d'intervention
directe sur le thalamus (injection, électrocoagulation)," *Rev.
neurol.*, 81:78–81.

Bell, E., and L. J. Karnosh (1949). "Cerebral Hemispherectomy," *J.
Neurosurg.*, 6:285–293.

Bettag, W. (1961). "Possibilités et limites des interventions centrales
sur le système thalamique dans les cas de douleurs irréductibles.

Étude basée sur les observations de 60 thalamotomies practiquées à differents niveaux," *Excp. Med. Int. Congr. Series,* 36:63–64 F.

———— and P. Rottgen (1961). "L'hemi-spasme facial et l'action thérapeutique de la destruction du centre médiothalamique," *Excp. Med. Int. Congr. Series,* 36:64–65 F.

Bettag, W., and T. Yoshida (1960). "Über stereotaktischen Schmerzoperationen," *Acta Neurochir.* (Vienna), 8:299–317.

Biemond, A. (1956). "The Conduction of Pain above the Level of the Thalamus Opticus," *Arch. Neurol. Psychiat.* (Chicago), 75:231–244.

Birkenfeld, R., and R. G. Fisher (1963). "Successful Treatment of Causalgia of Upper Extremity with Medullary Spinothalamic Tractotomy. Case Report and Review of the Literature," *J. Neurosurg.,* 20:303–311.

Bishop, G. H. (1962). "Anatomical, Physiological, and Psychological Factors in Sensation of Pain," in *Neural Physiopathology,* ed. R. Grenell (New York: Hoeber Med. Div., Harper and Sons) pp. 95–133.

Bohm, N. (1960). "Chordotomy for Intractable Pain due to Malignant Disease," *Acta psychiat.* (Kbh.), 35:145–155.

Bok, S. T. (1928); quoted by W. Noordenbos (1959).

Bonhöffer, K. (1928). "Klinische anatomische Beiträge zur Pathologie des Sehhügels und der Regio subthalamica," *Mschr. Psychiat. Neurol.,* 67:253–271.

Bonica, J. J. (1954). *The Management of Pain* (Philadelphia: Lea and Febiger).

Borellini, A. (1948). "Considerazioni sulle cordotomie posteriori nel trattamento delle paralisi spastiche," *Minerva Med.* (Turin), 39:539.

Bowsher, D. (1957). "Termination of the Central Pain Pathway in Man: The Conscious Appreciation of Pain," *Brain,* 80:606–622.

———— (1959). "The Anatomy of Thalamic Pain," *J. Neurol. Neurosurg. Psychiat.,* 22:81–82.

———— (1960). "The Terminal Distribution of the Pathways Subserving Pain," *J. Neurol. Neurosurg. Psychiat.,* 23:351.

Bressan, G. C., C. Cerciello, A. Fusco, and G. Pappalardo (1956). "Le cordotomie posteromediali nella cura delle paralisi spastiche," *Arch. Ortop.* (Milan), 69:223–237.

Brihaye, J., and J. Rétif (1961). "Comparaison des résultats obtenus par la cordotomie antérolatérale au niveau dorsal et au niveau cervical: A propos de 109 observations personnelles," *Neurochirurgie,* 7:258–277.

Brodal, A. (1948). *Neurological Anatomy in Relation to Clinical Medicine* (Oxford: Clarendon Press).

Browder, B., and J. P. Gallagher (1948). "Dorsal Chordotomy for Painful Phantom Limb," *Ann. Surg.*, 128:456–469.

Brower, B. (1933). "Centrifugal Influence on Centripetal System in the Brain," *J. nerv. ment. Dis.*, 77:621–627.

Campanini, T., and C. De Risio (1962). "Sul problema del 'dolore di origine centrale.' Osservazioni ed ipotesi suggerite da un caso clinico," *Sist. nerv.*, 14:382–386.

Carbonin, S. (1961). "Topectomia postcentrale per membro fantasma doloroso (MFD)," *Min. neurochir.*, 5:11–14.

Carreras, M., and F. Visintini (1965). "Fisiopatologia delle sensibilità somatiche," *Riv. Pat. nerv. ment.* (Florence), XV° Congresso Naz. della Soc. Ital. Neurol., pp. 1–83.

Cassinari, V., L. Infuso, and C. A. Pagni (1963a). "Some Experiences with Stereotaxic Surgery of Pain," *Excp. Med. Int. Congr. Series,* 60:121–123.

——— (1963b). "Prospettive attuali della chirurgia stereotassica del dolore," in *Atti del Simposium Int. Terapia di Blocco delle Sindromi Dolorose,* Venice, May 21–25 (Vicenza: Tip. Consonni), pp. 192–198.

Cassinari, V., C. A. Pagni, L. Infuso, and F. Marossero (1964). "La chirurgia stereotassica dei dolori incoercibili. Esperienza personale a proposito di 20 casi," *Sist. nerv.*, 16: 17–28.

Constans, J. P. (1960). "Chirurgie frontale de la douleur," *Acta Neurochir.* (Vienna), 8:251–281.

Cooper, I. S., L. L. Bergmann, and A. Caracalos (1963). "Anatomic Verification of the Lesion Which Abolishes Parkinsonian Tremor and Rigidity," *Neurology*, 13:779–787.

Crawford, A. S. (1947). "Medullary Tractotomy for Relief of Intractable Pain in Upper Levels," *Arch. Surg.* (Chicago), 55:523–529.

——— (1960). "Medullary Spinothalamic Tractotomy for High Intractable Pain," *J. Maine med. Ass.*, 51:233–235.

——— and R. S. Knighton (1953). "Further Observations on Medullary Spinothalamic Tractotomy," *J. Neurosurg.*, 10:113–121.

Dandy, W. E. (1933). "Physiological Studies following Extirpation of the Right Cerebral Hemisphere in Man," *Bull. Johns Hopk. Hosp.*, 53:31–51.

David, M., J. Talairach, and H. Hécaen (1947). "Étude critique des interventions neuro-chirurgicales actuellement pratiquées dans le traitement de la douleur," *Sem. Hôp.* (Paris), 23:1651–1655.

Davison, C., and W. Schick (1935). "Spontaneous Pain and Other Subjective Disturbances," *Arch. Neurol. Psychiat.* (Chicago), 34: 1204–1237.

Déjerine, J., and G. Roussy (1906). "La syndrome thalamique," *Rev. Neurol. fasc.*, 12:521–532.

D'Errico, A. (1950). "Intramedullary Spinothalamic Tractotomy," *J. Neurosurg.*, 7:294–298.

Dimitri, and Balado; quoted by M. David, *et al.* (1947).

Dogliotti, A. M. (1937). "Trattamento del dolore nei tumori," *Minerva Med.* (Turin), 28:455–461.

———— (1938). "First Surgical Sections, in Man, of the Lemniscus Lateralis (Pain-Temperature Path) at the Brainstem, for the Treatment of Diffused Rebellious Pain," *Anesth. et Analg.*, 17:143–145.

Drake, C. G., and K. G. McKenzie (1953). "Mesencephalic Tractotomy for Pain—Experience with Six Cases," *J. Neurosurg.*, 10:457–462.

Ebin, J. (1949). "Combined Lateral and Ventral Pyramidotomy in Treatment of Paralisis Agitans," *Arch. Neurol. Psychiat.* (Chicago), 62:27–47.

Echols, D. H., and J. A. Colclough (1947). "Abolition of Painful Phantom Foot by Resection of the Sensory Cortex," *J. Amer. med. Assoc.*, 134:1476–1477.

Elsberg, C. A. *Surgical Diseases of the Spinal Cord, Membranes, and Nerve Roots* (London: Lewis and Co.), 1941, 598 pp.

Erickson, T. C., W. J. Bleckwenn, and C. N. Woolsey (1952). "Observations on the Post-Central Gyrus in Relation to Pain," *Trans. Amer. neur. Ass.*, pp. 57–59.

Façon, E., N. Wertheim, and E. Mestes (1960). "Syndrome d'inattention spatiale avec douleurs d'origine corticale. Étude anatomo-clinique," *Rev. neurol.*, 102:61–74.

Fajersztain, J. (1895); quoted by W. Noordenbos (1959).

Falconer, M. A. (1949). "Intramedullary Trigeminal Tractotomy and Its Place in the Treatment of Facial Pain," *J. Neurol. Neurosurg. Psychiat.*, 12:297–311.

———— (1953). "Surgical Treatment of Intractable Phantom Limb Pain," *Brit. med. J.*, 1:299–304.

———— (1955); quoted by J. C. White and W. H. Sweet (1955).

Feld, M., and J. Pecker (1951). "Essais de cordotomie postérieure dans les paraplégies spasmodiques. Application sur syndrome paraplégique de Little," *Rev. neurol.*, 82:542–543.

Foerster, O. (1927). *Die Leitungsbahnen des Schmerzgefühls und die chirurgische Behandlung der Schmerzzustande* (Berlin: Urban und Schwarzenberg).

———— quoted by R. Garcin (1937).

———— and O. Gagel (1932). "Die Vorderseitenstrangdurchschneidung beim Menschen," *Z. ges. Neurol. Psychiat.*, 138:1–92.

Franceschelli, N., and C. Clivio (1948). "La cura chirurgica delle paralisi spastiche," *Minerva Med.* (Turin), 39:539.

Frazier, C. H., F. H. Lewy, and S. N. Rowe (1937). "The Origin and

Mechanism of Paraoxysmal Neuralgic Pain and the Surgical Treatment of Central Pain," *Brain*, 60:44–51.

French, L. A. (1958). "High Cervical Chordotomy," *Mississippi Doctor*, 35:231–232.

Fulton, J. F. (1951). *Physiology of the Nervous System* (New York: Oxford Univ. Press).

Garcin, R. (1937). "La douleur dans les affections organiques du système nerveux central," *Rev. neurol.*, 68: 105–153.

―――― (1957). "La douleur dans les affections du système nerveux central (thalamus, région bulbo-protubérantielle)," in *La douleur et les douleurs*, ed. Th. Alajouanine (Paris: Masson), 199–213.

―――― and J. Lapresle (1954). "Syndrome sensitif de type thalamique et à topographie cheiro-orale per lésion localisée du thalamus," *Rev. neurol.*, 90:124–129.

Gardner, E., and H. M. Cuneo (1945). "Lateral Spinothalamic Tract and Associated Tracts in Man," *Arch. Neurol. Psychiat.* (Chicago), 53:423–430.

Gardner, W. J., L. J. Karnosch, C. C. McClure, and A. K. Gardner (1955). "Residual Function following Hemispherectomy for Tumor and for Infantile Hemiplegia," *Brain*, 78:487–502.

Glees, P. (1953). "The Central Pain Tract," *Acta Neuroveg.* (Vienna), 7:160–174.

―――― (1961). *Experimental Neurology* (Oxford: Clarendon Press).

―――― and R. A. Bailey (1951). "Schichtung und Fasergrösse des Tractus spinothalamicus des Menschen," *Mschr. Psychiat. Neurol.*, 122:129–141.

Gobbel, W. G., and G. W. Liles (1945). "Efferent Fibers of the Parietal Lobes of the Cat (Felis domesticus)," *J. Neurophysiol.*, 8:257–266.

Goldschneider, A. (1898); quoted by W. Noordenbos (1959).

Grant, F. C., (1948). "Complications accompanying Surgical Relief of Pain in Trigeminal Neuralgia," *Amer. J. Surg.*, 75:42–47.

―――― R. A. Groff, and F. H. Lawy (1940). "Section of the Descending Spinal Root of the Fifth Cranial Nerve," *Arch. Neurol. Psychiat.* (Chicago), 43:498–509.

Grant, F. C., and L. H. Weinberger (1941). "Experiences with Intramedullary Tractotomy. IV Surgery of the Brainstem and Its Operative Complications," *Surg. Gynec. Obstet.*, 72:747–754.

Greif, quoted by R. Garcin (1937).

Guidetti, B. (1950). "Nevralgia essenziale del trigemino. Sezione del tratto trigeminale discendente bulbare secondo il metodo di Siöqvist," *Sist. nerv.*, 2:247–257.

Guillain, G., and I. Bertrand (1932). "Lésion atrophique symétrique des circonvolutions pariétales ascendantes et des circonvolutions occipitales," *Ann. med.* 31:35–58.

Guillaume, J. (1942). "Myélotomie postérieure pour algies post-zostériennes et moignons douloureux avec membres fantômes. Remarques physiopathologiques," *Rev. neurol.*, 74:317–319.

––––––– and G. Mazars (1949). "Remarques à propos de la cordotomie cervicale haute," *Rev. neurol.*, 81:770–777.

Guillaume, J., and J. Sigwald (1947). *Diagnostic neuro-chirurgical* (Paris: Presses Universitaires de France).

Guillaume, J., I. Bertrand, and G. Mazars (1945). "Un cas de moignon douloureux traité par myélotomie. Etude électroencéphalographique et considérations physiopathologiques." *Rev. neurol.*, 77:145.

Guiot, G. (1964), personal communication.

––––––– and S. Forjaz (1947). "La tractotomie mésencéphalique par voie sous-temporale," *Rev. neurol.*, 79:733–740.

Gutiérrez-Mahoney, de, C. G. (1944). "The Treatment of Phantom Limb by Removal of Post-Central Cortex," *J. Neurosurg.*, 1:156–162.

––––––– (1948). "The Treatment of Painful Phantom Limb—A Follow-up Study," *Surg. Clin. N. Amer.*, 28:481–483.

Haghbart, K. R., and D. I. B. Kerr (1954). "Central Influences on Spinal Afferent Conduction," *J. Neurophysiol.*, 17:295–307.

Hamby, W. B., B. M. Shinners, and I. A. Marsh (1948). "Trigeminal Tractotomy: Observations on 48 Cases," *Arch. Surg.* (Chicago), 57:171–177.

Hankinson, J. (1962). "Neurosurgical Aspects of Relief of Pain at the Cerebral Level," in *The Assessment of Pain in Man and Animals*, ed. C. A. Keele and R. Smith (Edinburgh and London: Livingstone), pp. 135–143.

––––––– G. W. Pearce, and G. Rowbotham (1960). "Stereotactic Operations for the Relief of Pain," *J. Neurol. Neurosurg. Psychiat.*, 23:352.

Hassler, R. (1960). "Die zentrale Systeme des Schmerzes," *Acta neurochir.* (Vienna), 8:353–423.

––––––– and T. Riechert (1959). "Klinische und anatomische Befunde bei stereotaktischen Schmerz-operationen im Thalamus," *Arch. Psychiat. Nervenkr.*, 200:93–122.

Head, H., and G. Holmes (1911). "Sensory Disturbances from Cerebral Lesions," *Brain*, 34:102–254.

Hécaen, H. (1957). "L'asymbolie à la douleur" in *La douleur et les douleurs*, ed. Th. Alajouanine (Paris, Masson), pp. 259–265.

Hécaen, H., J. Talairach, M. David, and M. B. Dell (1949). "Coagulations limitées du thalamus dans les algies du syndrôme thalamique. Résultats thérapeutiques et physiopathologiques." *Rev. neurol.*, 81:917–931.

Hoff, H., K. Pateisky, and T. Wanko (1953). "Thalamus und Schmerz," *Acta Neuroveg.* (Vienna), 7:277–300.

Hoffmann, W. (1933). "Thalamussyndrom auf Grund einer kleinen Läsion," *J. Psychol. Neurol.* (Leipzig), 54:362–374.

Holbrock, T. J., and C. G. de Gutiérrez-Mahoney (1947). "Diffusion of Painful Stimuli over Segmental, Infrasegmental, and Suprasegmental Levels of the Spinal Cord," *Fed. Proc.*, 6:131.

Horrax, G. (1946). "Experiences with Cortical Excisions for the Relief of Intractable Pain in the Extremities," *Surgery*, 20:593–602.

―――― and E. Lang (1957). "Complications of Chordotomy," *Surg. Clin. N. Amer.*, 37:849–854.

Hyndman, O. R. (1942). "Lissauer's Tract Section. A Contribution to Chordotomy for the Relief of Pain. Preliminary Report," *J. int. Coll. Surg.*, 5:394–400.

―――― and C. van Hepps (1939). "Tumor of the Thalamus. A Ventriculographic Entity," *Arch. Surg.* (Chicago), 39:792–797.

Imber, I. (1930). "I tumori del talamo ottico," *Morgagni*, 72:1887–1904.

Johnson, F. H. (1954). "Experimental Study of Spinoreticular Connections in the Cat," *Anat. Rec.*, 118:316.

Jouvet, P., C. Lapras, G. Tusini, and P. Wertheimer (1960). "Mise en evidence chez l'homme au cours d'enregistrements stéréotaxiques thalamiques d'un contrôle central des afférences somesthésiques," *Acta neurochir.* (Vienna), 8:287–292.

Jung, R. (1959). "Neurophysiologische und neurologiche Aspekte zentraler Schmerzzustände." Erste Europäischen Neurochirurgenkongress. *Acta neurochir. Vorausdruck der Referate*, pp. 11–15.

Karplus, I. P., and A. Kreidl (1914). "Ein Beitrag zur Kenntnis der Schmerzleitung im Rückenmark," *Pflüg. Arch. ges. Physiol.*, 158:275–287.

―――― (1925). "Zur Kenntnis der Schmerzleitung im Rückenmark. II Mitteilung," *Pflüg. Arch. ges. Physiol.*, 207:134–139.

Keegan, J. J. (1947). "Dermatome Hypalgesia Associated with Posterolateral Herniation of Lower Cervical Intervertebral Disc," *J. Neurosurg.*, 4:115–139.

Kendall, D. (1939). "Some Observations on Central Pain," *Brain*, 62:253–273.

Kerr, F. W. L. (1961). "Structural Relation of the Trigeminal Spinal Tract to Upper Cervical Roots and the Solitary Nucleus in the Cat," *Exp. Neurol.*, 4:134–148.

Klemme, R. (1949). "Relief of Pain by Section of the Spinothalamic Tract at the Level of the Olivary Nucleus," *J. int. Coll. Surg.*, 12:754–756.

Kletzkin, M., and E. A. Spiegel (1952). "Spinal Pain Conduction by Chains of Short Neurons," *Fed. Proc.*, 11:83.

Laine, E., M. Fontan, Delandtsheer, and Desfontaines (1952). "Étude d'un série d'hémispherectomie pour hémiplégie infantile," *Rev. neurol.*, 86:344–350.

Laine, E., and C. Gros (1956). *L'hémispherectomie* (Paris: Masson).

Lapresle, J., and G. Guiot (1953). "Étude des résultats éloignées et en particulier des sequelles neurologiques à type de 'douleur centrale' dans 8 cas de cordotomie antérolatérale pour coxarthrose," *Sem. Hop.* (Paris), 29:2189–2198.

Laspiur, D. R. (1956). "Estereotaxis (en relacion a dos casos operados de sindrome talàmico vascular)," *Arch. Instit. de Neurocir.* pp. 97–113.

Le Beau, J. (1953). *Psycho-chirurgie et fonctions mentales* (Paris: Masson).

———, S. Daum, and S. Forjaz (1948). "Les tractotomies trigéminales dans le traîtement des névralgies faciales," *Brasil Méd. cir.*, 10:331–344.

Leriche, R. (1937). "Neurochirurgie de la douleur," *Rev. neurol.*, 68:317–342.

——— (1949). *La chirurgie de la douleur* (Paris: Masson).

Lewin, W., and C. G. Phillips (1952). "Observations on Partial Removal of the Postcentral Gyrus for Pain," *J. Neurol.*, 15:143–147.

Lhermitte, J. (1933). "Physiologie des ganglions centraux. Les corps striés. La couche optique. Les Formations sous-thalamiques," in *Traité de physiologie normale et pathologique*, ed. G. H. Roger and L. Binet (Paris: Masson), IX, 357–402.

——— and J. de Ajuraguerra (1935). "Syndrome hemialgique fruste par rammollissement pariétal," *Rev. neurol.*, 64:204–210.

Lhermitte, J., and P. Puech (1946). "L'algo-hallucinose des amputes. Traitement par la résection du névrome, l'infiltration de la chaîne sympathique, une double myélotomie postérieure, la résection du lobale pariétal supérieur," *Rev. neurol.*, 78:33–35.

Livingston, R. B. (1959). "Central Control of Receptors and Sensory Transmission Systems," in *Handbook of Physiology*, ed. J. Field, H. W. Magoun, and V. E. Hall (Washington: Am. Physiol. Soc.), I, 741–760.

Macchi, G., and F. Angeleri (1957). "Anatomia sperimentale dei sistemi a proiezione diffusa dell'encefalo," in *Atti del Convegno di Parma*, November 23–24, 1957, pp. 41–80.

Macchi, G., G. Dalle Ore, and R. Da Pian (1964). "Reperti anatomici in soggetti operati di talamotomia stereotassica," *Sist. nerv.*, 16:193–223.

Mansuy, L., J. Lecuire and L. Acassat (1944). "Technique de la myélotomie commissurale postérieure," *J. Chir.* (Paris), 60:206–213.

Mark, H. V., F. R. Ervin, and T. P. Hackett (1960). "Clinical Aspects of Stereotactic Thalamotomy in the Human. Part 1. The Treatment of Chronic Severe Pain," *Arch. Neurol.*, 3:351–367.

Mark, H. V., F. R. Ervin, and P. I. Yakovlev (1962). "The Treatment of Pain by Stereotaxic Methods." *Conf. neurol.*, 22:238–245.

——— (1963). "Stereotactic Thalamotomy. III Verification of Anatomical Lesion Site in the Human Thalamus," *Arch. Neurol.*, 8:528–538.

Marshall, J. (1951). "Sensory Disturbances in Cortical Wounds with Special Reference to Pain," *J. Neurol. Neurosurg. Psychiat.*, 14: 187–204.

May, W. P. (1906). "The Afferent Path. The Conduction of Painful Impulses in the Spinal Cord," *Brain*, 29:782–784.

Maspes, P. E., and C. A. Pagni (1965). "Studio critico degli interventi sterotassici eseguiti a livello talamico per il trattamento dei dolori incoercibili," *Riv. Pat. nerv. ment.* (Florence), Congresso Naz. della Soc. Ital. Neurol. pp. 1–154.

Mazars, G., A. Pansini, and J. Chiarelli (1960). "Coagulation du faisceau spino-thalamique et du faisceau quinto-thalamique par stéréotaxie. Indications. Résultats." *Acta neurochir.* (Vienna), 8:324–326.

Mazars, G., R. Rogé, and A. Pansini (1960). "Stereotactic Coagulation of the Spinothalamic Tract for Intractable Trigeminal Pain," *J. Neurol. Neurosurg. Psychiat.*, 23:352.

Mehler, W. R. (1957). "The Mammalian 'Pain Tract' in Phylogeny," *Anat. Rec.*, 127:332.

——— (1966). "Some Observations on Secondary Ascending Afferent Systems in the Central Nervous System," in *Pain*, eds. R. S. Knighton, P. R. Dumke (Boston, Mass.: Little, Brown and Co.), pp. 11–32.

———, M. E. Feferman, and W. J. Nauta (1956). "Ascending Axon Degeneration following Anterolateral Chordotomy in the Monkey," *Anat. Rec.*, 124:332–333.

Melzack, R., and F. P. Haugen (1957); quoted by R. Hassler (1960).

Mikula, F., J. Siroky, and B. Zapletal (1959). "Le traitement des crises gastralgiques par la tractotomie mésencephalique bilaterale et ses complications auditives inattendues," *Rev. oto-neuro-oftal.* (Buenos Aires), 31:456–463.

Miserocchi, E. (1951). "Le cordotomie (tractotomie spinali)," *Chirurgia*, 6:519–538.

Monnier, M. (1955). "Les résultats de la coagulation du thalamus chez l'homme (noyau ventro-postérieur)," *Acta neurochir.* (Vienna), suppl. 3, 291–307.

——— and R. Fischer (1951). "Stimulation électrique et coagulation thérapeutique du thalamus chez l'homme (névralgies faciales)," *Confin. neurol.* (Basel), 11:282–286.

Morello, G. (1962). "La chirurgia del dolore," in *Atti delle Giornate Mediche Triestine,* (Trieste: Casa Editrice Giuliana), pp. 149– 160.

Morin, F., H. G. Schwarz, and J. L. O'Leary (1951). "Experimental Study of the Spinothalamic and Related Tracts," *Acta psychiat.* (Kbh.), 26:371–396.

Moruzzi, G., and H. W. Magoun (1949). "Brainstem Reticular Formation and Activation of the EEG," *Electroenceph. clin. Neurophysiol.,* 1:455–473.

Mountcastle, V. B., and T. P. S. Powell (1959). "Neural Mechanisms Subserving Cutaneous Sensibility, with Special Reference to the Role of Afferent Inhibition in Sensory Perception and Discrimination," *Bull. Johns Hopk. Hosp.,* 105:201–232.

Nathan, P. W. (1956). "Reference of Sensation at the Spinal Level," *J. Neurol. Neurosurg. Psychiat.,* 19:88–100.

Nicolesco, M. (1924), quoted by J. de Ajuraguerra (1937).

Noica, D., and M. Balls (1935). "Contribution à la physiologie de la couche optique," *Encéphale,* 2:554–561.

Noordenbos, W. (1959). *Pain. Problems Pertaining to the Transmission of Nerve Impulses Which Give Rise to Pain* (Amsterdam: Elsevier Publ. Co.).

Obrador, S. (1956), quoted by E. Laine and C. Gros (1956).

——— and G. Bravo (1960). "Thalamic Lesions for the Treatment of Facial Neuralgias," *J. Neurol. Neurosurg. Psychiat.,* 23:351– 352.

Obrador, S., R. Carrascosa, and M. Sevillano (1961). "Observaciones sobre la estimulaciòn y lesiòn talàmica en mano fantasma dolorosa," *Rev. esp. Oto-neuro-oftal.,* 20:149–153.

Obrador, S., G. Dierssen, and R. Ceballos (1957). "Consideraciones clinicas, neurologicas y anatomicas sobre el llamado dolor talàmico (con motivo de dos casos personales)," *Acta neurol. lat.-amer.,* 3:58–77.

Olivecrona, H. (1947a). "Notes on the Surgical Treatment of Migraine," *Acta med. scandin.,* 128:229–238 (suppl. 196).

——— (1947b). "The Surgery of Pain," *Acta psychiat.* (Kbh.), suppl. 46.

Oliver, L. C. (1949). "Surgery in Parkinson's Disease. Division of Lateral Pyramidal Tract for Tremor," *Lancet,* 1:910–913.

——— (1950). "Surgery in Parkinson's Disease. Complete Section of the Lateral Column of the Spinal Cord for Tremor," *Lancet,* 1:847– 848.

Olszewski, J. (1950). "On the Anatomical and Functional Organization of the Spinal Trigeminal Nucleus," *J. comp. Neurol.*, 92:401–413.

———— (1954). "The Cytoarchitecture of the Human Reticular Formation," in *Brain Mechanisms and Consciousness*, ed. E. D. Adrian, F. Bremer, and H. H. Jasper (Oxford: Blackwell), pp. 54–80.

Osàcar, E. M., A. E. Meyer, and I. Jakab (1961). "A Histologically Verified Bilateral Anterolateral Chordotomy without Cutaneous Sensory Loss. A Case Report," *Acta neurochir.* (Vienna), 9:524–537.

Pagni, C. A. (1966). Discussion to F. R. Erwin, C. E. Brown, V. H. Mark: "Striatal Influence on Facial Pain," *Confin. neurol.* (Basel), 27:88–89.

Pagni, C. A., E. Wildi, G. Ettorre, L. Infuso, F. Marossero, and G. P. Cabrini (1965). "Anatomic Verification of Lesion Which Abolished the Tremor and Rigor in Parkinsonism," *Confin. neurol.* (Basel), 26:291–294.

Pearson, A. A. (1952). "Role of Gelatinous Substance of Spinal Cord in Conduction of Pain," *Arch. Neurol. Psychiat.* (Chicago), 68:515–529.

Pecker, J., and J. Le Beau (1957). "Cinq observations d'allachestésie, trouble sensitif d'un type particulier observé après cordotomie," *Rev. neurol.*, 96:62–68.

Peele, T. L. (1954) *The Neuroanatomical Basis for Clinical Neurology* (New York: McGraw-Hill).

Pellegrini, G., and I. Papo (1962). "Il sistema neurovegetativo nella patogenesi del dolore e dello shock," in *La chirurgia del simpatico* (symposium) (Rome: EMES), pp. 65–136.

Penfield, W., and R. Boldrey (1937). "Somatic Motor and Sensory Representation in the Cerebral Cortex of Man as Studied by Electrical Stimulation," *Brain*, 60:389–443.

Penfield, W., and H. H. Jasper (1954). *Epilepsy and Functional Anatomy of the Human Brain* (Boston: Little, Brown).

Petit-Dutaillis, D. (1937). "A propos de l'indication de la cordotomie (cordotomie au lieu d'élection et cordotomie cervicale haute)," *Rev. neurol.*, 68:347–352.

————, R. Messimy, and L. Berges (1953). "La psychochirurgie des algies irréductibles. Étude basée sur 57 cas," *Sem. Hôp.* (Paris), 29:3893–3903.

Petit-Dutaillis, D., R. Messimy, and H. Feld (1950). "Troubles sensitifs et sensorielles après ablation préfrontale chez l'homme," *Rev. neurol.*, 83:23.

Pieri, G. (1951). "Contributi clinici alla mielotomia," *Chir. ital.*, 5:515–517.

Pierre, Marie, quoted by R. Garcin (1937).

Poggio, G. F., and V. B. Mountcastle (1960). "A study of the Functional Contributions of the Lemniscal and Spinothalamic Systems to Somatic Sensibility. Central Nervous Mechanisms of Pain," *Bull. Johns Hopk. Hosp.*, 106:266–316.

Pool, J. L. (1946). "Posterior Chordotomy for Relief of Phantom Limb Pain," *Ann. Surg.*, 124:386–391.

Putnam, T. J. (1933). "Treatment of Athetosis and Dystonia by Sections of Extrapyramidal Motor Tracts," *Arch. Neurol. Psychiat.*, (Chicago), 29:504–521.

——— (1934). "Myelotomy of the Commissure—A New Method of Treatment for Pain in the Upper Extremities," *Arch. Neurol. Psychiat.* (Chicago), 32:1189–1193.

——— (1938). "Results of Treatment of Athetosis by Section of Extrapyramidal Tracts in the Spinal Cord," *Arch. Neurol. Psychiat.* (Chicago), 39:258–275.

——— (1940). "Treatment of Unilateral Paralysis Agitans by Section of the Lateral Pyramidal Tract," *Arch. Neurol. Psychiat.* (Chicago), 44:950–976.

Puusepp, L. (1930); quoted by O. Antonucci (1938).

Quarti, M., and H. Terzian (1954). "L'emisferectomia nel trattamento delle emiplegie infantili," *Chirurgia*, 9:339–350.

Ramón y Cajal, S. (1899). *Textura del sistema nervioso del hombre y de los vertebrados* (Madrid: Imprenta y libreria de Nicolas Moya). Tomo I, 566 pp., Tomo II, 1209 pp.

Rand, R. W. (1960). "Further Observations on Lissauer Tractolysis," *Neurochirurgia*, 3:151–168.

Ranson, S. W., and S. L. Clark (1957). *The Anatomy of the Nervous System. Its Development and Function* (Philadelphia: Sanders).

Rasmussen, A. T. (1945). *The Principal Nervous Pathways* (London: Macmillan).

——— and W. T. Peyton (1948). "The Course and Termination of the Medial Lemniscus in Man," *J. comp. Neurol.*, 88:411–424.

Ray, B. S., and H. G. Wolff (1945). "Studies in Pain: 'Spread of Pain.' Evidence on Site of Spread within the Neuraxis of Effects of Painful Stimulations," *Arch. Neurol. Psychiat.* (Chicago), 53:257–261.

Riddoch, G. (1938). "The Clinical Features of Central Pain," *Lancet*, 234:1093–1098, 1150–1156, 1205–1209.

——— and M. Critchley (1937). "La physiopathologie de la douleur d'origine centrale," *Rev. neurol.*, 68:77–104.

Riechert, T. (1961). "Méthodes stéréotaxiques dans la chirurgie de la douleur," *Excp. Med. Int. Congr. Series*, 36:34–35 F.

Rizzatti, E. (1939). "Cordotomia posterior medialis nella paraplegia spastica tipo Little," *Policlinico, Sez. prat.*, 46:1897–1901.

Roeder, F., and H. Orthner (1961). "Erfahrungen mit stereotaktischen Eingriffen. III Mitteilung. Über zerebrale Schmerzoperationen, insbesondere mediale Mesencephalotomie bei thalamischer Hyperpatie und bei Anaesthesia dolorosa," *Confin. neurol.* (Basel), 21:51–97.

Rose, J. E., and V. B. Mountcastle (1959). "Touch and Kinestesis," in *Handbook of Physiology*, ed. J. Field, H. W. Magoun, and V. E. Hall (Washington: Am. Physiol. Soc.), I, 387–429.

Rossi, G. F., and A. Brodal (1957). "Terminal Distribution of Spinoreticular Fibers in the Cat," *Arch. Neurol. Psychiat.* (Chicago), 78:439–453.

Rossi, G. F., and A. Zanchetti (1957). "The Brainstem Reticular Formation. Anatomy and Physiology," *Arch. ital. Biol.* (Pisa), 95: 199–435.

Roulhac, G. E. (1953). "High Cervical Chordotomy," *Surgery*, 34:288–295.

Roussy, G. (1907). *La couche optique (étude anatomique, physiologique et clinique* (Paris: G. Steinheil), 349 pp.

Rowbotham, G. F. (1938). "Treatment of Pain in the Face by Intramedullary Tractotomy," *Brit. med. J.*, 2:1073–1076.

———— (1961). "A Case of Intractable Pain in the Head and Face Associated with Pathological Changes in the Optic Thalamus," *Acta neurochir.* (Vienna), 9:1–8.

Sasaki, K. (1938). "Über die Wirkung der Chordotomie auf Spontangangren," *Arch. klin. Chir.*, 192:448–461.

Sager, quoted by R. Garcin (1937).

Scarff, J. E. (1950). "Unilateral Prefrontal Lobotomy for the Relief of Intractable Pain. Report of 58 Cases with Special Consideration of Failures," *J. Neurosurg.*, 7:330–336.

Schürmann, K. (1953). "Über das Spätergebnis der chirurgischen Behandlung extrapyramidalen Bewegungsstörungen und paraplegischer Zustände," *Dtsch. Z. Nervenheilk*, 169:24–28.

———— (1957). "Die Chirurgie der extrapyramidalen Hyperkinesen," in *Handbuch der Neurochirurgie*, ed. H. Olivecrona and W. Tonnis (Berlin: Springer Verlag), VI, 58–136.

Schuster, P. (1936); quoted by R. Garcin (1937) and by E. A. Walker (1938).

Schwartz, H. G. (1950). "Neurosurgical Relief of Intractable Pain," *Surg. Clin. N. Amer.*, 30:1379–1389.

———— and J. L. O'Leary (1941). "Section of the Spinothalamic Tract in the Medulla with Observations on the Pathway for Pain," *Surgery*, 9:183–193.

———— (1942). "Section of the Spinothalamic Tract at the Level of the Inferior Olive," *Arch. Neurol. Psychiat.* (Chicago), 47:293–304.

Serra, A., and V. Neri (1936). "Die elektro-chirurgische Unterbrechung der Zentralbahnen des V Paares am lateralen ventralen Rand des Pons Varoli als esters Behandlungsversuch von hartnätigen Neuralgien des Trigeminus durch tumoren des Schadelbasis," *Zbl. Chir.*, 63:2248–2251.

Sicard, J. A., J. Hauguenau, and R. Wallich (1927). "Cordotomie latérale antérieure dans une algie paroxystique du moignon. Isothermognosie," *Bull. Soc. méd Hôp.* (Paris), 51:1219–1221.

Sie Pek Giok (1956); quoted by W. Noordenbos (1959).

Siöqvist, O. (1938). "Studies on Pain Conduction in the Trigeminal Nerve. A Contribution to the Surgical Treatment of Facial Pain," *Acta psychiat.* (Kbh.), suppl. 17, 139.

——— (1949). "Surgical section of pain tracts and pathways in the spinal cord and brain stem." *IVe Congr. neurol.*, 1:119–132.

——— (1950). "La section chirurgicale des cordons et des voies de la douleur dans la moelle et le tronc cérébral," *Rev. neurol*, 83:38–40.

Smyth, G. E., and K. Stern (1938). "Tumors of the Thalamus. A Clinicopathological Study," *Brain*, 61:339–374.

Sokolianski, G. G., and E. F. Kulkowa (1938). "Über die Rolle des Sehhügels in der Klinik von Störungen der Sensibilität. Zur Frage der Genese der thalamischen Hyperpathie," *Zbl. ges Neurol. Psychiat.*, 91:215–216.

Spiegel, E. A., M. Kletzkin, E. G. Szekely, and H. T. Wycis (1954). "Role of Hypothalamic Mechanisms in Thalamic Pain," *Neurology* (Minneapolis), 4:739–751.

Spiegel, E. A., and H. T. Wycis (1953). "Mesencephalotomy in Treatment of Intractable Facial Pain," *Arch. Neurol. Psychiat.* (Chicago), 69:1–13.

——— (1962). Stereoencephalotomy. Part II: *Clinical and Physiological Application* (New York: Grune and Stratton), p. 504.

——— and H. Freed (1952). "Stereoencephalotomy. Thalamotomy and Related Procedures," *J. Amer. Med. Ass.*, 148:446–451.

Sprague, J. M., and H. Ha (1964). "The Terminal Fields of Dorsal Root Fibers in the Lumbosacral Spinal Cord of the Cat, and the Dendritic Organization of the Motor Nuclei," in *Organization of the Spinal Cord*, ed. J. C. Eccles and J. P. Schadé (Amsterdam: Elsevier Pub. Co.), pp. 120–154.

Starzl, T. E., and H. W. Magoun (1951). "Organization of the Diffuse Thalamic Projection System," *J. Neurophysiol.*, 14:133–146.

Stewart, W. A., and R. B. King (1961). "A New Ascending Spinal Trigeminal Neural Pathway," *Surg. Forum*, 12:386–388.

——— (1963). "Fiber Projections form the Nucleus Caudalis of the Spinal Trigeminal Nucleus," *J. comp. Neurol.*, 121:271–286.

BIBLIOGRAPHY

Stewart, W. A., W. L. Stoops, and R. B. King (1963). "Trigeminal Dorsal Root Reflex," *Surg. Forum*, 14:405–407.

Stewart, W. A., W. L. Stoops, P. R. Pillone, and R. B. King (1964). "An Electrophysiologic Study of Ascending Pathways from Nucleus Caudalis of the Spinal Trigeminal Nuclear Complex," *J. Neurosurg.*, 21:35–48.

Stone, T. T. (1950). "Phantom Limb Pain and Central Pain. Relief by Ablation of Portion of Posterior Central Cerebral Convolution," *Arch. Neurol. Psychiat.* (Chicago), 63:739–748.

Sugar, O., and P. Bucy (1951). "Postherpetic Trigeminal Neuralgia," *Arch. Neurol. Psychiat.* (Chicago), 65:131–145.

Sweet, W. H., V. H. Mark, and H. Hamlin (1960). "Radiofrequency Lesions in the Central Nervous System of Man and Cat, Including Case Reports of Eight Bulbar Pain-Tract Interruptions," *J. Neurosurg.*, 17:213–225.

Szentàgothai, J. (1964). "Propriospinal Pathways and their Synapses," in *Organization of the Spinal Cord*, ed. J. C. Eccles and J. P. Schadé (Amsterdam: Elsevier Publ. Co.), pp. 155–177.

Talairach, J., H. Hécaen, M. David, M. Monnier, and J. de Ajuraguerra (1955); quoted by E. A. Spiegel and H. T. Wycis (1962).

Talairach, J., P. Tournoux, and J. Bancaud (1960). "Chirurgie pariétale de la douleur," *Acta neurochir.* (Vienna), 8:153–250.

Taren, J. A., and E. A. Kahn (1962). "Anatomic Pathways Related to Pain in Face and Neck," *J. Neurosurg.*, 19:116–121.

Testut, L. (1943). *Anatomia Umana*, Libro quinto, Sistema Nervoso Centrale (Torino, Unione Tipografico-Editrice Torinese), 716 pp.

Torvik, A. (1959). "Sensory Motor and Reflex Changes in Two Cases of Intractable Pain after Stereotactic Mesencephalic Tractotomy," *J. Neurol. Neurosurg. Psychiat.*, 22:299–305.

Tovi, D., G. Schisano, and B. Liljeqvist (1961). "Primary Tumor of the Region of the Thalamus," *J. Neurosurg.*, 18:730–740.

Tower, S. S., D. Bodian, and H. Rowe (1941). "Isolation of Intrinsic and Motor Mechanism of the Monkey's Spinal Cord," *J. Neurophysiol.*, 4:388–397.

Turnbull, F. (1939). "Chordotomy for Thalamic Pain: A Case Report," *Yale J. Biol. Med.*, 11:411–414.

Vincent, C., quoted by J. C. White and W. H. Sweet (1955).

Voris, H. C. (1957). "Variations in the Spinothalamic Tract in Man," *J. Neurosurg.*, 14:55–60.

Walker, E. A. (1938). "The Anatomical Basis of the Thalamic Syndrome," *J. belge Neurol. Psychiat.*, 38:69–95.

———— (1940). "The Spinothalamic Tract in Man," *Arch. Neurol. Psychiat.* (Chicago), 43:284–298.

———— (1942a). "Mesencephalic Tractotomy. A Method for the Relief of Unilateral Intractable Pain," *Arch. Surg.* (Chicago), 44:953–962.

———— (1942b). "Somatotopic Localization of Spinothalamic and Secondary Trigeminal Tracts in Mesencephalon," *Arch. Neurol. Psychiat.* (Chicago), 48:884–889.

———— (1950). "The Neurosurgical Treatment of Intractable Pain," *Lancet*, 70:279–282.

———— (1955). "El significado del talamo," *Rev. Neuro-psiquiat.*, 18:131–150.

Walshe, E. O. (1959). *Physiology of the Nervous System* (London: Longmans, Green), p. 563.

Watts, J. W., and W. Freeman (1948); quoted by T. T. Stone (1950).

Wertheimer, P., and J. Lecuire (1953). "La myélotomie commissurale postérieure. A proposo de 107 observations," *Acta chir. belg.*, 52:568–574.

Wertheimer, P., and L. Mansuy (1949). "Quelques tentatives neurochirurgicales centrales dans le traîtement des douleurs irréductibles," *Rev. neurol.*, 81:401–408.

Wertheimer, P. and J. Sautot (1949). "Les résultats de la myélotomie commissurale postérieure. A propos de 69 observations," *Concours med.*, 71:413–414.

White, J. C. (1941). "Spinothalamic Tractotomy in the Medulla Oblongata. An Operation for the Relief of Intractable Neuralgias of Occiput, Neck, and Shoulder," *Arch. Surg.* (Chicago), 43:113–127.

———— (1962). "Evaluation of Operations for Relief of Pain," *Neurologia Medico-chirurgica*, 4:1–28.

✗ ———— (1963). "Anterolateral Chordotomy—Its Effectiveness in Relieving Pain of Non-malignant Disease," *Neurochirurgia*, 6:83–102.

✗ ———— and W. H. Sweet (1955). *Pain. Its Mechanisms and Neurosurgical Control* (Springfield, Ill.: Charles Thomas Publ.) p. 736.

Wilson, S. A. K. (1927). "Dysaesthesiae and Their Neural Correlates," *Brain*, 50:428–462.

Windle, W. F. (1926). "Non-bifurcating Nerve Fibers of the Trigeminal Nerve," *J. comp. Neurol.*, 40:229–240.

Winkler, C. (1917); quoted by W. Noordenbos (1959).

Wycis, H. T. (1961). Discussion to T. Riechert (1961). *Excp. Med. Int. Congress Series*, 36:35.

———— and E. A. Spiegel (1962). "Long-Range Results in the Treatment of Intractable Pain by Stereotaxic Midbrain Surgery," *J. Neurosurg.*, 19:101–107.

Zihen, T. (1899); quoted by W. Noordenbos (1959).

Zulch, K. J. (1960). "Schmerzbefunde nach operativen Eingriffen am Zentralnervensystem (Hemisphärektomie, olivare Traktotomie)," *Acta neurochir.* (Vienna), 8:282–286.

———— (1963). "Morphologische und klinische Typen," in *Die in-*

fantile Zerebralparesen, ed. K. Lindemann (Stuttgart: Georg Thieme Verlag), pp. 1–28.

———— and E. E. Schmid (1953). "Über die Schmerzarten und den Begriff der Hyperpathie," *Acta neuroveg.* (Vienna), 7:147–159.

SUBJECT INDEX

AUTHOR INDEX

189